Right Down Your Alley

The Beginners' Book of Bowling

Vesma Grinfelds
WIBC Hall-of-Famer Pro Bowler
Former NBC Clinician

Bonnie Hultstrand
Professor Emeritus, Physical Education
University of Idaho

WADSWORTH

✦

THOMSON LEARNING

Australia Canada Mexico Singapore Spain United Kingdom United States

WADSWORTH
THOMSON LEARNING

Publisher: Peter Marshall
Acquisition Editor: April Lemons
Assistant Editor: John Boyd
Editorial Assistant: Andrea Kesterke
Marketing Manager: Jennifer Somerville
Marketing Assistant: Mona Weltmer
Advertising Project Manager: Shemika Britt
Composition Buyer: Ben Schroeter
Print/Media Buyer: Robert King
Project Editor: Sandra Craig
Permissions Editor: Beth Zuber

Production Service: Carlisle Communications
Text Designer: Harry Voigt
Copy Editor: Chris Feldman
Illustrator: Terry Wolbers
Cover Designer: Harry Voigt
Cover Image: Getty Images
Cover Printer: Patterson Printing
Compositor: Carlisle Communications
Printer: Patterson Printing

Printed in the United States of America
1 2 3 4 5 6 7 06 05 04 03 02

For more information about our products, contact us at:
Thomson Learning Academic Resource Center
1-800-423-0563
For permission to use material from this text, contact us by:
Phone: 1-800-730-2214
Fax: 1-800-730-2215
Web: http://www.thomsonrights.com

Library of Congress Control Number
2002104173

Wadsworth/Thomson Learning
10 Davis Drive
Belmont, CA 94002-3098
USA

Asia
Thomson Learning
5 Shenton Way #01-01
UIC Building
Singapore 068808

Australia
Nelson Thomson Learning
102 Dodds Street
South Melbourne, Victoria 3205
Australia

Canada
Nelson Thomson Learning
1120 Birchmount Road
Toronto, Ontario M1K 5G4
Canada

Europe/Middle East/Africa
Thomson Learning
High Holborn House
50/51 Bedford Row
London WC1R 4LR
United Kingdom

Latin America
Thomson Learning
Seneca, 53
Colonia Polanco
11560 Mexico D.F.
Mexico

Spain
Paraninfo Thomson Learning
Calle/Magallanes, 25
28015 Madrid, Spain

ISBN 0-534-56031-8

Preface

Throughout this book, we authors (one a former professional bowler and national clinician and the other a former teacher and bowling coach) have attempted to combine all of the newest and proven techniques, equipment, and teaching/learning concepts that are presently being used by bowlers, coaches, and teachers across the country. Our approach to bowling includes a high degree of natural feeling involvement in the movement pattern. Complimenting this naturalness is the integration of efficient movement principles for accuracy and consistency in delivery and ball roll.

In this day of high technology, bowling has changed a great deal. We find manufacturers seeking the ultimate bowling balls, lanes, pins, and lane conditions. Therefore, *Right Down Your Alley: The Beginners' Book of Bowling* includes a section on how these twenty-first century changes affect delivery, ball roll, and aiming and some of the adjustments that may be used to be effective in today's environment.

We include everything a beginning bowler, regardless of age or ability, needs to know about the game of bowling in order to be successful. We have also taken a bold step forward in presenting materials for left-handed bowlers as well as right-handed bowlers. We hope that this text gives each reader a better understanding of the elements involved in the game of bowling and will enhance your enjoyment and performance in the number one indoor participant sport in the country.

In addition to the text, the accompanying Instructor's Manual/Test bank includes a variety of teaching/learning concepts, tools, teaching cues, and games to assist in the learning bowling. The IM/TB also includes chapter objectives, detailed chapter outlines, and a variety of test questions, including multiple choice, true/false, and fill-in-the-blank.

Vesma Grinfelds
Bonnie Hultstrand

Acknowledgments

The authors wish to extend their sincere gratitude to the many friends who have helped make this book possible. We especially thank Kathy Clark and Dorothy Zakrajsek for the constant encouragement and patient assistance in editing the manuscript; Corinne Lyle for the unending hours in assisting with the editing and formatting of the manuscript; Dzintars Grinfelds for his computer assistance and photography supervision; Lloyd Terrell, assisted by Greg Harris and Bordon Chin of RTL Photography, and Eric Risberg for providing the fine photographs; Sea Bowl in Pacifica, CA, and the Classic Bowling Center for graciously providing the bowling facilities; Virginia Norton and her teaching expertise; Tracy Castro, Heidi Kindorf, Stephanie Yee, Jennifer Jones, Sean Johnson, Phillip Campit, Steve Villanueva, Dzintars Grinfelds, Jim McEntee, Teresa Fletcher, Rodney Garrick, Marianne Petroni, Maxine Anderson, Ruth Noll, Marie Papia, and Dominic Papia, who so willingly gave of their time to be subjects for the photographs; Rod Ross and Terry Leong, who provided insight into the rapidly changing bowling environment, drilling techniques, and modern game; and Teresa Fletcher, who assisted in obtaining the "models" and caring for the details. We would also like to express our appreciation to the former National Bowling Council for providing us with many of the illustrations and information. We are deeply appreciative to our editor, April Lemons, for her assistance and insight during this revision. We would also like to thank the reviewers for their comments and suggestions: Ginny Leath, North Carolina State University; Enrico Odorico, Macomb Community College; Frank Ormond, North Carolina State University; David Stodden, Auburn University; and Katherine Davis, Slippery Rock University. To all of you, we are deeply indebted!

Contents

Basic Bowling

Understanding the Basics

On the surface, the game of bowling appears quite simple. The bowler takes an approach, rolls a fairly heavy ball down a 60-foot lane, and with two attempts tries to knock down the ten wooden pins placed in a triangular fashion at the end of the lane. However, as the bowler delves into the mechanics of bowling, he or she finds a much more complicated game. Hopefully, in the next few chapters of this text the mysteries of successful bowling will be uncovered so each person may find that measure of success and knowledge that are sought.

It is true that each bowler establishes his or her own style. However, truly successful bowlers seem to have many attributes in common: (1) They all have a smooth, flowing approach and delivery; (2) they all have excellent timing, balance, and flexibility during the approach and delivery; (3) their swing and approach is absolutely consistent on each delivery; (4) they have complete concentration, poise, and confidence; and (5) each has developed a system of adjustment to assist in compensating for outside forces where bowlers have little control, such as varying lane conditions. These above attributes do not just happen. They are practiced, thought through, and then grooved to the extent of becoming automatic.

The key to success in bowling lies in knowing the game inside and out, and being able to groove the entire approach, swing, and delivery where consistency is an absolute.

In the following chapters, we intend to present all of the information necessary for a bowler to achieve his or her potential. The material presented has been tried and proven by the best in the world.

Features of the Ball, Pins, and Lanes

Understanding ball, lane, and pin composition, and the dimensions of each, will aid the bowler in grasping the mechanical and mathematical concepts involved in bowling.

Bowling Ball

Bowling balls range from 8 to 16 pounds in weight and are constructed of hard rubber, synthetic plastic, urethane, or reactive resin materials. The number of finger holes in the ball vary from two to five, but the ball with three finger holes is the most common. The finger holes in the bowling balls are drilled at different sizes, widths, and angles to fit the grip and size desired by the individual bowler (see Chapter 2).

No matter what the weight, the ball measures approximately 27 inches in circumference and about 8½ inches in diameter (Figure 1.1).

Bowling Pins

Bowling pins are made of durable materials, usually hard rock maple covered by a thin plastic coating. Many bowling establishments are replacing these maple pins with synthetic pins that tend to last longer. These pins are 15 inches in height and 15 inches in circumference around the belly of the pin. The diameter is approximately 4¾ inches through the widest part (Figure 1.1). According to the American Bowling Congress (ABC), pins may be no lighter than 3 pounds 6 ounces, and no heavier than three pounds ten ounces. Furthermore, the set of pins in service at an establishment must all be of the same weight. On the bottom of the pin there is a nylon cap to protect it from wear and tear. Taking these specifications into

consideration, it is interesting to note than a pin will topple when it moves 10 degrees off its vertical axis.

There are ten pins set on the lane in a 36-inch equilateral triangle, with each pin around the perimeter of the triangle and across the rows spread 12 inches apart, center to center (Figure 1.2).

Interesting note: In examining the ball dimensions in relation to the pins, it is found that a single pin left standing could be contacted by the ball anywhere within a 22-inch area. It should also be noted that a ball cannot pass directly between two adjoining pins without contacting one or both of them (Figure 1.1).

The pins are numbered from front to back, always starting from left and going to the right. Before proceeding, the reader must memorize the pins by their correct number (Figure 1.3).

Figure 1.1
Relative dimensions of ball and pins.

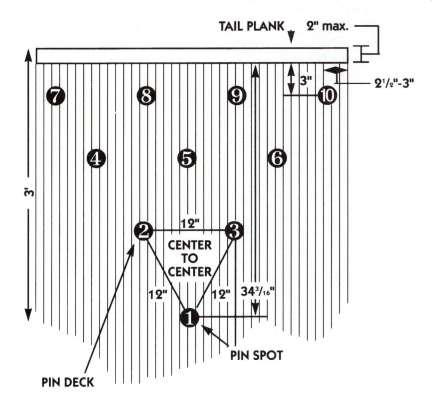

Figure 1.2
In an ABC regulation bowling lane, the pins are arranged in a 36-inch equilateral triangle. Each pin is 12 inches from the adjacent pin, center to center. (Courtesy of former NBC)

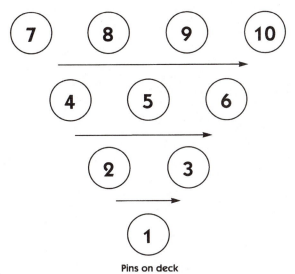

Figure 1.3
The pins are numbered from left to right.

Lane Features and Dimensions

In order for a bowler to understand the bulk of material yet to be presented in this text, it is imperative to understand and be able to identify the different parts of the lane and its dimensions.

The bowling area is divided into four segments—the approach, the lane, the pin deck, and the pit area.

The Approach

The **approach** is the area found toward the back of the lane where bowlers take their steps and swing prior to the delivery of the ball. The approach is made up of laminated boards that are a little over an inch in width and about 4 inches thick set on end. These boards match the 39 boards that make up the lane in front of the approach area.

Usually on this approach, a bowler may identify three rows of dots extending parallel to the foul line. These dots are known as locator dots and are used by bowlers in finding their proper stance. The first row of locator dots can be found 2 to 3 inches behind the foul line. The other two rows are found 12 and 15 feet, respectively, from the foul line (Figure 1.4). The dots are equally placed 5 boards apart and the center dot is in the center of the approach, which corresponds to the 20th board in the center of the lane.

The Lane

The **lane** is the area in front of the approach and foul line where the ball rolls to encounter the pins. The width of the lane is approximately 42 inches, made up of 39 laminated boards slightly over an inch in width plus a narrower filler board usually found somewhere between the edge board and first arrow on the left.

The length of the lane from the foul line to the center of the head pin is 60 feet (Figure 1.4). In the traditional lanes, the first one-third of the lane, plus the outside board, and the area under the pins is constructed of hard maple that is extremely durable. The remainder of the lane to the head pin is constructed of pine. Since pine is much softer and contains more grain, it assists the bowling ball in

"grabbing" the lane, resulting in greater hooking action. *Note:* There are also many synthetic lanes made of laminates that have a wood-like appearance. The dimensions and markings on these lanes are the same as on wood lanes.

The Pin Deck and Pit Area

On the lane area, we find 7 large markings placed in an inverted V formation, known as **target arrows.** These target arrows have special significance to each bowler as they help bowlers to focus on a specific target while delivering the ball, a procedure known as **spot bowling.** These target arrows are located 15 feet from the foul line with the center arrow on the 20th board. Just as on the approach, these arrows are also spaced 5 boards apart and are in perfect alignment (Figure 1.5). For right handers, this means that the 3rd arrow from the right corresponds with the 15th board, the second arrow is on the 10th board, and the

---

Self Evaluation Questions

1. How many boards make up a bowling lane?

2. How many boards apart are the locator dots placed?

3. What is the minimum length of a bowling approach?

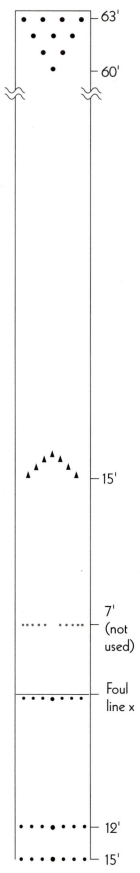

Figure 1.4
Relative distance of lane and approach markings from the foul line.

first arrow is located on the 5th board (Figure 1.5).

***Please note:* Left handers** number these target arrows from left to right. For left handers, this means that the 3rd arrow from the left corresponds to the 15th board, the 2nd arrow from the left is on the 10th board, and the 1st arrow

on the left is on the 5th board (Figure 1.5).

Halfway between the foul line and the target arrows, there is a row of dots called the spots. These spots are *not* lined up with the other locator dots or target arrows and are of little or no use to the average bowler. The spots are of value to higher average bowlers, those who are extremely

nearsighted, or those who have physical handicaps.

The area of the lane where the pins are set is called the **pin deck** (Figure 1.6). It is approximately 36 inches in depth and is made of hardwood and durable synthetic materials to take the wear and tear of falling and flying pins.

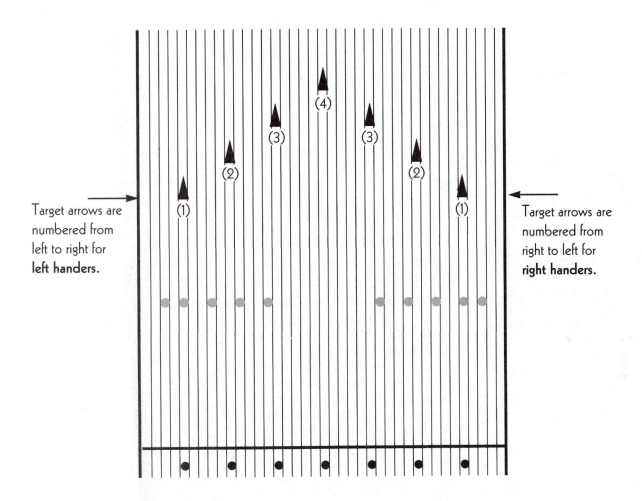

Target arrows are numbered from left to right for **left handers.**

Target arrows are numbered from right to left for **right handers.**

Figure 1.5
The target arrows are aligned with the locator dots at the foul line and are placed on every 5th board. ***Note:*** The spots between the foul line and target area *do not* line up with the target arrows and the locator dots. These spots are *not* used for our purposes. (Courtesy of former NBC)

Self Evaluation Questions

1. How many boards apart are the target arrows?

2. Are they in line with the locator dots on the approach?

3. How many boards make up the width of a lane?

4. How far is it from the foul line to the head pin?

Figure 1.6
The markings on the pin deck denote where the pins will be placed.

To the sides of the pin deck are side partitions called **kickbacks** that help contain the pins and assist pin action on the pin deck. These kickbacks span the entire area from opposite the head pin to the rear cushion found above the pit area.

The **pit area** is approximately 4¾ inches below the surface of the pin deck and extends another 30 inches back to the cushion. This area is recessed in order to catch the pins before they have a chance to bounce back out on the lane. It usually contains a movable belt that carries the ball back to the ball return and the pins into the automatic pinsetter.

Etiquette and Safety

There are many commonly accepted rules of **etiquette** that everyone should follow upon entering the bowling establishment. By using common sense and following these basic rules of etiquette, we will assist the management in keeping maintenance costs down, be respected and appreciated by others on the lanes, and help make the game of bowling pleasant and safe for all.

Basic Rules of Etiquette and Safety

- Before stepping onto the lane, check to make sure the bowlers on the adjoining lanes are not in their stance or taking their approach. The rule is: **Only one person on the approach at a time.** If you both step up on the approach at the same time, **yield to the person on the right** (Figure 1.7).
- Bowling is a sport that requires intense concentration. Therefore, refrain from disturbing any bowler in his or her approach. Loud noises and constant movement are very distracting to all.
- Restrict your body English and confine your elation or disappointment to your own lane or within yourself. Kicking the ball return or other equipment doesn't help anyone.
- After you have delivered the ball, walk straight back and step off the approach while waiting for the return of the ball (Figure 1.8).
- Take a *reasonable* amount of time while on the approach area but think of others. Many people become irritated if they have to wait too long for someone else.
- Use only *your* ball, towel, resin, and other equipment unless you have permission to borrow someone else's.
- Keep refreshments out of the bowler's settee area. Spilled liquids present problems to all bowlers (Figure 1.9).
- Be prepared to bowl when it is your turn. Plan your absences from the lane so no one will have to wait for you to return.

Figure 1.7
A bowler on the right takes his or her turn first.

Figure 1.8
No matter how pleased you are with the result, confine your elation to your own lane and walk straight back from the foul line.

Figure 1.9
Food and drink should remain behind the settee area.

- Change into your bowling shoes before entering the bowling area. This will keep the area free from mud, water, and dirt that may be picked up by bowler's shoes and carried onto the lanes.
- Refrain from blaming someone else or equipment for your mistakes. More than likely it is your fault when things go wrong.
- Refrain from giving advice to others unless they ask for your help.
- Make sure the ball sweep is up before you deliver the ball (Figure 1.10).
- Avoid lofting the ball. This is damaging to the lanes as well as distracting to others (Figure 1.11).
- Avoid wearing long skirts, long floppy pants, floppy sleeves, or jewelry which may get tangled during the approach and cause a mishap.

Figure 1.10
When the sweep is down in front of the pins, do *not* bowl.

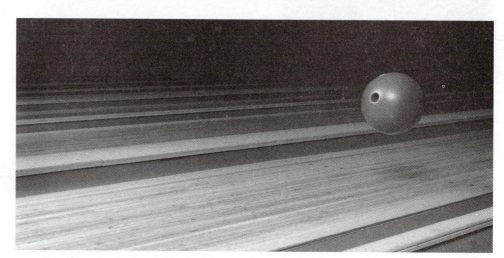

Figure 1.11
Do not loft the ball. This lofted delivery is 7 feet forward of the foul line and has not yet touched the lane.

- When lifting your bowling ball back from the rack, to avoid pinched fingers and back strain, place both hands on the ball (one on each side), bend your knees, and lift by straightening the legs (Figure 1.12).
- Avoid going beyond the foul line (Figure 1.13).
- Respect the rights and privacy of others by *not* using your cell phone during bowling (Figure 1.14).

By following these simple rules, bowling will be more enjoyable to all. Remember the basic rule of good manners: **Be Considerate of Others.**

Figure 1.12
The proper way to remove a ball from the ball rack, minimizing the chances of hand or finger injury.

Figure 1.14
Respect the rights and privacy of others by *not* using your cell phone during bowling.

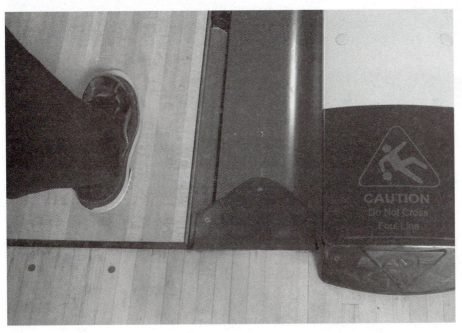

Figure 1.13
Do not step over the foul line.

In a Nutshell:

- In order to become a good bowler you must groove the approach, the swing, and the delivery. This can only be accomplished through good practice.
- The bowling pins are set in a precise 36 inch equilateral triangle; are spaced 12 inches apart from center to center; and are numbered from left to right.

- The head pin is located on the 20th board and is 60 feet from the foul line.
- The approach is a minimum of 15 feet in length and has 3 sets of locator dots. These locator dots are used to assist the bowler in exact foot placements on his or her stance and approach.
- The locator dots are spaced 5 boards apart with the center dot on the 20th board. The dots and boards are always counted from the outside edge of the lane toward the center. For right handers, this is from right to left. For left handers, this is from left to right.
- The target arrows used for aiming in spot bowling are 15 feet in front of the foul line. They are also spaced 5 boards apart and are in direct line with the locator dots on the approach.
- The basic rule of etiquette and safety involves being considerate of others.
- Remember the basic rule of good manners:
  Be Considerate of Others.

2

Preparing for Action

Selection of Proper Equipment

Proper selection of equipment is essential for bowling success. Two basic equipment needs are (1) a pair of bowling shoes that are properly fitted and (2) a well-fitted ball.

Bowling Shoes

The **bowling shoes** rented at a bowling establishment are dual-purpose shoes that can be used by right or left handers because both the left and right soles are made of sliding material. When renting shoes, make sure that they fit comfortably and will slide at the end of the approach. Care must be taken when purchasing a pair of bowling shoes because they are made differently for left- and right-handed bowlers. The soles of most higher quality shoes are constructed to give one foot some traction, while giving the other foot a sole for sliding purposes. **For right handers,** sliding at the foul line when

delivering the ball is done on the left foot. In order to ensure a smooth slide, the left sole is usually made of leather. The right foot is used for traction so the right sole of the shoe is usually rubber with a leather tip. **For left handers,** sliding at the foul line when delivering the ball is done on the right foot. Therefore, the right sole is usually made of leather to ensure a smooth slide. The left foot used for traction will find a shoe with a rubber sole with a leather tip (Figure 2.1).

Bowling Ball

To provide consistency, it is desirable for an individual to purchase a **bowling ball** and have it professionally selected and fitted. If this is not possible, then care must be exercised when selecting a "house" ball. It should be heavy enough to add stability to the swing, and yet not so heavy that it causes the shoulder to drop. Keep in mind, a heavier ball will have less deflection when it hits the pins, resulting in better pin coverage.

Figure 2.1
Soles of bowling shoes are not all identical.

Figure 2.2
Different types of grips:
(a) Conventional;
(b) Fingertip; (c) Semi-fingertip.

(a)

(b)

(c)

We recommend the following guidelines:

- For children under twelve, use a bowling ball that is 1 pound for every 10 pounds of body weight. This should come close to eight-year-olds using an 8-pound ball; a ten-year-old using a 10-pound ball, and so on.
- Most beginning women bowlers should be able to start with an 11 or 12-pound ball, and as they progress they can move up to a heavier ball.
- Most beginning male bowlers should be able to start with a 14- or 15 pound ball. Eventually, they may also want to move to a heavier ball.

After attending to the weight of the ball, the next consideration is hand and finger fit. The two most important factors to consider are the size of the thumb and finger holes and the span from the thumb to the fingers.

The thumb should comfortably and snugly fit into the thumb hole. It should come out of the hole with a little resistance but without popping. If the thumb hole is too large, many problems will arise by trying to grip the ball much too tightly with the thumb joint. The finger holes should fit the fingers fairly snug and should allow the fingers to come out smoothly and without resistance.

The second important element in obtaining a proper fit is determining the span or distance between the thumb and the fingers according to the preferred grip—**conventional, fingertip,** or **semi-fingertip** (Figure 2.2).

The most common grip that has the shortest span is the **conventional grip.** Most "house" balls are drilled with this grip which potentially allows the bowler to develop a high degree of accuracy and ball control. The second most popular grip with the largest span is the **fingertip grip.** It is used by consistent and highly skilled bowlers looking to achieve a higher degree of hook power and pin action. The **semi-fingertip** span is slightly wider than the conventional yet shorter than the fingertip and is potentially useful for a bowler to increase the lift imparted at the point of release.

Most novice and intermediate bowlers use the conventional grip (Figure 2.3). In order to find the proper span for the **conventional**

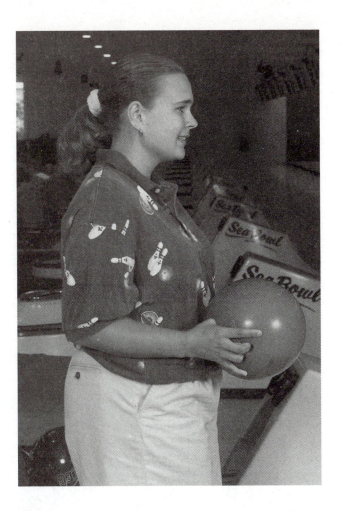

Figure 2.3
Conventional grip.

Figure 2.4
Fingertip grip.

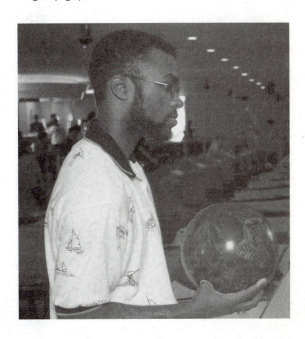

grip, place the thumb all the way into the thumb hole. Making sure the wrist remains straight, extend the fingers across the span area of the ball. The lines on the second knuckle of your middle finger should exceed the edge of the finger hole closest to the thumb by about 1/4 of an inch.

The second most popular bowling grip is the **fingertip.** Since the span is wider in this fingertip grip than in the conventional grip, measurement is made by using the first joint of the fingers instead of the second joint as in the conventional grip. To find the proper fit for the fingertip ball, place the thumb all the way in the thumb hole and extend the fingers over the surface of the ball. The line of the first joint will land right in the middle of the fingerhold. If the ball fits correctly with the thumb and fingers in the ball, the second knuckle should be sticking up in the air slightly and forming a little triangle

(Figure 2.4). If it is flat against the surface of the ball, the span is too long and the evidence will be burnt fingertips or excessive calluses. To ensure a properly drilled fingertip ball, a professional driller in a reputable pro shop should be sought.

Conventional vs. Fingertip Discussion:

In comparing the advantages and disadvantages of the aforementioned conventional and fingertip grips, one finds that neither is perfect. Of the two, the conventional grip probably helps develop greater accuracy. The major disadvantage of the conventional grip is that the hooking action is only minimal because so much of the hand is inside the ball. The thumb comes out first, but, due to the compactness of the fingers, not enough time elapses for proper hand action to take place. This results in reduced hooking action with less pin carry.

The fingertip ball may be less accurate than the conventional grip but has a greater pin carry due to an increased hooking action. This greater hooking action is a result of greater lift and more revolutions that can be imparted on the ball with the wider span.

The third type of grip, called the **semi-fingertip,** was designed to combine the advantages of both the conventional and fingertip—the control and accuracy of the conventional and the extra hooking action of the fingertip. The span is equidistant between the two first joints of the fingers. This particular grip has been found unsatisfactory primarily because the fingers cannot bend at the location between the two joints. This causes the fingers to grip the back of the hole and often causes discomfort to the bowler. It has not been as successful as originally anticipated and is not highly recommended.

Self Evaluation Questions

1. What are two important considerations in properly fitting a bowling ball?

2. What are the three basic grips found in bowling balls?

3. How would you find the proper span for a conventional grip?

Holding the Ball

In order to obtain maximum accuracy and consistency, it is absolutely essential that the hand position be held constant throughout the stance, swing, and delivery. This action will assist in allowing the ball to be delivered exactly the same on each ball delivery.

The most effective ball delivery is the one that results in the ball hooking slightly at the end of the ball roll into the strike pocket or proper selected key pin. This delivery is called a **hook ball** and is highly desirable since there is a off center ball rotation which allows the ball to enter the pins at a slight angle minimizing deflection and maximizing "digging" action (Figure 2.5A and 2.5B)

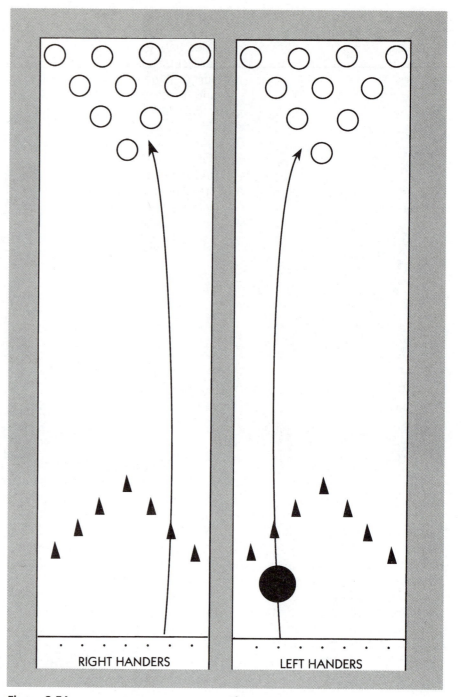

Figure 2.5A
Right Handers—The path of a hook ball due to the fingers lifting off the center of the ball from the 4 o'clock position. The result is a counter-clockwise rotation.

Figure 2.5B
Left Handers—The path of a hook ball of a left hander where fingers lift off the center of the ball from the 8 o'clock position, resulting in a clockwise rotation.

This entire action, in turn, results in maximum **pin carry** by splattering the pins more sideways as the ball continues to roll into the 5 pin in the center of the triangle. The ball rotation imparted on the ball is merely an automatic result of the fingers applying upward pressure or lift on the ball from the 4 o'clock position by right handers and the 8 o'clock position for left handers, both being applied off the center of the ball. *Note:* It is the authors' belief that due to the hook ball's superiority in pin action over the straight ball, all bowlers should learn from the very beginning the hook ball delivery. Therefore, all further discussion will be surrounding the roll of the hook ball and its effective use.

In finding the correct hand position for the *hook ball,* visualize the ball with a clock face on it. The center of the clock face is between the finger and thumb holes of the ball. Standing in the appropriate position with the ball supported in the non-bowling hand (Figure 2.6), the right-handed bowler places the thumb and finger holes in a 10 and 4 o'clock position, respectively (Figure 2.7). The left-handed bowler places the thumb at 2 and fingers at 8 o'clock (Figure 2.8).

By turning the ball face now slightly to the side while maintaining the 10 and 4 o'clock (right handers) or the 2 and 8 o'clock (left handers) positions, the fingers and thumb are inserted and the wrist will be found firm and straight in relation to the bowler's forearm (Figures 2.7 and 2.8).

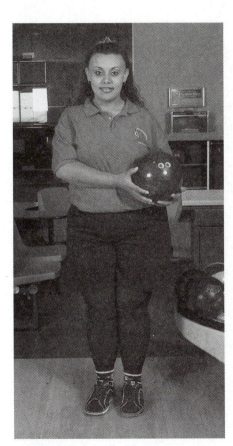

Figure 2.6
When taking the stance position, the ball is held in the non-bowling hand.

Figure 2.7
Right Handers—The 10–4 o'clock position used to deliver a hook ball.

Figure 2.8
Left Handers—The 2–8 o'clock position used to deliver a hook ball.

Note: Good control is associated with gripping the ball firmly. Spread the two outside fingers apart and press downward against the surface of the ball with the tips of the fingers. This will help keep the wrist firm to create maximum control at delivery.

Self Evaluation Questions

1. Why is a hook ball recommended?

2. In what position are the thumb and fingers placed in the ball to roll a hook ball?

3. How can you firm the wrist while gripping the ball?

Aiming in Bowling

There are two main ways to aim in bowling—pin bowling and spot bowling. **Pin bowling,** used primarily by novice bowlers, is little more than sighting at the pins at the end of the lane. **Spot bowling,** which has been found to be the most successful and accurate method, is aiming at the target arrows 15 feet in front of the foul line.

Of the two, spot bowling is the preferred method of aiming due to the consistency it promotes. Consistency is very important in the game of bowling, and aiming is no exception. In spot bowling for **right-handed bowlers,** the second and third target arrows from the right will be the constant targets (Figure 2.9A). For **left-handed bowlers,** it will be the second and third arrows from the left (Figure 2.9B).

What are the advantages of **spot bowling?** First of all, it is undeniably easier to hit a target 15 feet away than one 60 feet away. Secondly, all bowling lanes are constructed the same so the bowler has a uniform

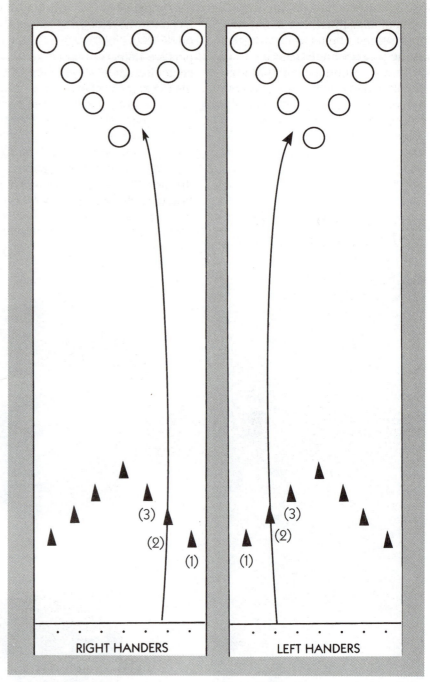

Figure 2.9A
Right Handers—During spot bowling, the second arrow from the right becomes the prime target.

Figure 2.9B
Left Handers—During spot bowling, the second arrow from the left becomes the prime target.

place to focus the eyes and make rational adjustments. Spot bowling also creates a better approach form by keeping a more balanced finishing position. Finally, it assists with the follow-through motion of the release by giving the bowler something to reach toward with the extended delivery arm.

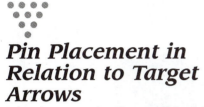

Pin Placement in Relation to Target Arrows

It has been previously established that the pins are setting in a perfect 36-inch triangle on the pin deck. We have also noted that the lane is made up of 39 boards with the head pin centered on the 20th board. Keep in mind the pins are 12 inches apart from the center to center. Also remember that the target arrows on the lane and all of the locator dots on the approach are spaced 5 boards apart.

Note: Since the pins are 5 1/2 boards apart, it should be noted that the target arrows *do not* line up with the pins. Therefore, for **right-handed bowlers,** the head pin is located on the 20th board; the 2 pin is near the 26th board; and the 3 pin is setting near the 14th board (Figure 6.1). With this in mind, one sees that the right hander's pocket for a **"perfect" strike** is halfway between the head pin and 3 pin (1–3) or the 17th board.

The Brooklyn pocket for right handers is between the head pin and the 2 pin. **Remember:** The right side of the lane is for right handers and they count boards and target arrows starting from the right-hand channel toward the left. The left side of the lane is for left handers and they count boards and target arrows starting from the left-hand edge. The **left hander's "perfect" strike pocket** is the 1–2 pocket. Therefore, if the head pin is on the 20th board, the 2 pin would be near the 14th board from the left. Therefore, counting the boards from left to right, the 1–2 pocket is on the 17th board. Crossing over to the 1–3 pocket would be the 23rd board (Figure 2.10).

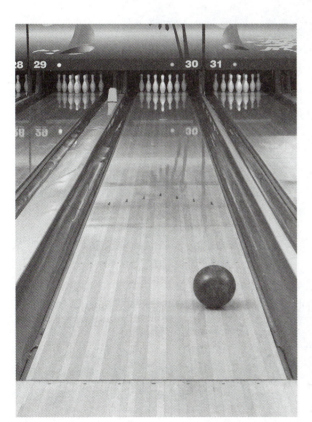

Figure 2.10A
Right Handers. To achieve a perfect strike, the ball must cross the 17th board at an angle. Delivering the ball across the second arrow helps to accomplish this.

Figure 2.10B
Left Handers. To achieve a perfect strike, the ball must cross the 17th board at an angle. Delivering the ball across the second arrow helps to accomplish this.

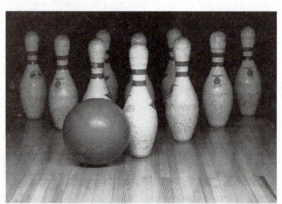

Self Evaluation Questions

1. How many boards apart are the pins?

2. Do they line up with the target arrows and locator dots?

3. On which board do we find the following:

    a. Head pin

    b. 2 pin

    c. 3 pin

    d. 1–3 pocket

    e. 1–2 pocket for left handers

Perfect Strike Pin Action

It is every bowler's dream to roll a perfect game of 300, which is stringing twelve strikes in a row. Such an accomplishment is elusive at best. To obtain the **perfect strike,** in comparison to a "sloppy" or "lucky" strike, it is an absolute necessity for the ball to roll into that perfect strike pocket at the proper angle.

Right Handers: In a perfect strike, the ball only contacts 4 pins on its way through to the pit area—the 1, 3, 5, and 9 pins. The rest of the pinfall is due to a chain reaction of falling pins. If the ball's angle of entry is exact, hitting the correct impact point on the head pin, the result will be the head pin falling into the 2 pin; the 2 pin falling to the 4; and the 4 pin hitting the 7 pin. This row of pins (1, 2, 4, 7) is called the "**accuracy line**" of pins. As a result of hitting the correct impact point on the 3 pin, it will fall in the opposite direction, taking out the 6 pin, with the 6 pin hitting the 10 pin. This line of pins (3, 6, 10) is called the "**carry line.**" The ball with its driving action should contact the 5 pin, which in turn falls into the 8 pin.

Finally, the ball itself hits the 9 pin (Figure 2.11A).

Left Handers: In a perfect strike, the ball only contacts four pins on its way through to the pit area—the 1, 2, 5, and 8 pins. The rest of the pinfall is due to a chain reaction of falling pins. If the ball's angle of entry is exact, hitting the correct impact point on the head pin, the result will be the head pin falling into the 3 pin; the 3 pin falling into the 6 pin; and the 6 pin falling into the 10 pin. This row of pins (1, 3, 6, 10) is known as the left hander's "accuracy line." As a result of hitting

the correct impact point on the 2 pin, the 2 pin will fall in the opposite direction taking out the 4 pin, and the 4 pin then takes out the 7 pin. This pin fall is called the "carry line." The ball contacts the 1, 2, 5, and 8 pins. The 5 pin takes out the 9 pin (Figure 2.11B).

This entire successive domino action results in a "perfect" strike. It is a result of the ball entering the pocket on the exact board, at the exact angle, with sufficient ball weight and enough roll to avoid undue ball deflection.

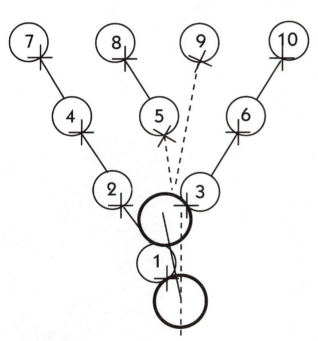

Figure 2.11A
Right Handers. The ball and pin action in a perfect strike. (Courtesy of former NBC)

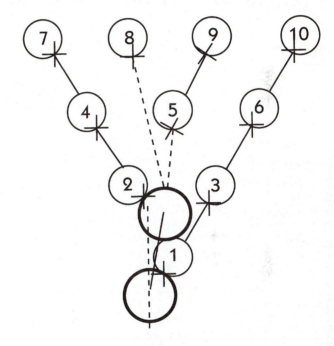

Figure 2.11B
Left Handers. The ball and pin action in a perfect strike. (Courtesy of former NBC)

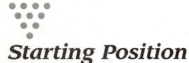

Starting Position

Now that we have a basic understanding of what our bowling ball is supposed to accomplish as it hits the pins, it is now time to examine possibly the most important part of one's bowling technique, the starting position on the approach.

Note: Since the four-step approach is the easiest approach to learn and in order to get some semblance of timing, rhythm, and a feeling for the movement of the ball, we will be presenting everything from a four-step basis.

In order to find a place on the approach as a **point of origin or starting position,** two questions must be answered: (1) How far from the foul line should the stance be taken to start the approach, and (2) on which dot or board should the feet be placed in order to roll the ball over the second target arrow?

To find the distance from the foul line, a bowler should go to the foul line and turn his or her back to the pins. The heels are placed in front of the locator dots (Figure 2.12). While keeping the eyes focused on the far wall, the bowler takes either three steps and a slide or four steps plus another half step toward the end of the approach area. The spot where the last foot ended will mark the correct starting distance from the line. This position may be adjusted slightly as need arises. Most bowlers of an average height and average temperament will end up around the 12 foot line.

The distance may vary from individual to individual due to:

(1) the length of the legs, (2) the height of the individual, and (3) the type of personality (e.g., the active person will take livelier and longer steps than the slow, easy-going person).

The second assessment that must be made concerns the lateral placement of the feet on the approach. The exact board from which a bowler should start is, again, somewhat individualistic because it depends upon the shoulder and hip width of the individual. The best measurement for a **right-handed** bowler is to stand far enough left on the approach so the right arm, hanging at the side, is in direct line with the target arrow, which is also the locator dots corresponding to the 10th board. In this position the bowler's hips and shoulders are

---

Self Evaluation Questions

1. What are the two impact points for a perfect strike? (right and left handers)

2. In the following diagram of the pins, show the ball and pin action for a perfect strike. (Indicate whether right- or left-handed)

Figure 2.12
To find the starting distance from the foul line, place heels two to three inches away from the foul line.

"square" to the aiming point. Looking down at the inside edge of the left shoe (right handers), note the exact location of the inside edge of that foot. This will be your starting position and should remain constant in order for you to gain accuracy and consistency (Figure 2.13A). The best measurement for a **left-handed bowler** is to stand far enough right on the approach so the left arm, hanging at the side, is in direct line with the target arrow corresponding to the 10th board from the left. In this position the bowler's hips and shoulders are "square" to the aiming point. Looking down at the inside edge of the right shoe (left handers), note the exact location of the inside edge of that foot. This will be your starting position and should remain constant in order for you to gain accuracy and consistency (Figure 2.13B).

In Preparing for Action We Have Now Found:

- The bowling ball should be the proper weight and fit.
- There are two main methods of aiming—pin bowling and spot bowling—but the most accurate and easiest to learn of the two is spot bowling.
- The ball only strikes 4 pins in a perfect strike. The remaining pins are a result of pin action and deflection.
- Proper foot placement for the stance point of origin is twofold:

(1) distance from the foul line and (2) lateral placement to line up the bowling arm with the second target arrow.

Right-handed bowlers only:
- Right-handed bowlers should wear right-handed player shoes.
- In order for a perfect strike to occur, the ball must enter the 1–3 pocket at an angle and be equidistant between the 1 and 3 pin.
- The pins are spaced approximately 5 1/2 boards apart so the 1–3 pocket is halfway between each of the pins or three boards to the right of the head pin, or the 17th board.
- In order to roll a hook ball, the ball is held with the thumb at the 10 o'clock position and the fingers at 4 o'clock.

Figure 2.13A
Right Handers—Check the exact location of the inside edge of the left foot in the stance position.

Figure 2.13B
Left Handers—Check the exact location of the inside edge of the right foot in the stance position.

- In spot bowling, the second and third target arrows from the right, found approximately 15 feet in front of the foul line, are the point of aim for right-handed bowlers.

Left-handed bowlers only:
- Left-handed bowlers should wear left-handed player shoes.
- In order for a perfect strike to occur, the ball must enter the 1–2 pocket at an angle and be equidistant between the 1 and 2 pin.

- The pins are spaced approximately 5 1/2 boards apart so the 1–2 pocket is halfway between each of the pins, or three boards to the left of the head pin, 17th board from the left.
- In order to roll a hook ball, the ball is held with the thumb at the 2 o'clock position and the fingers at 8 o'clock.
- In spot bowling, the second and third arrows from the left, found approximately 15 feet in front of the foul line, are the point of aim for left-handed bowlers.

Hints For Success

- While a partner supports the ball, place your thumb and fingers in it. Now place a pencil under the palm of your hand. If the finger span is correct, the pencil will not slide out easily (Figure 2.14).
- While the ball rests on a solid surface, insert your thumb and fingers. If it is a proper fit, a friend can tuck a little finger under the palm (Figure 2.15).

Self Evaluation Questions

1. How far back on the approach should you stand?

2. How do you measure this?

3. How do you know where your left foot should be placed in your stance?

4. How many steps are recommended for the approach?

Figure 2.14
Placing a pen or pencil under the palm is a way to check the span.

Figure 2.15
Inserting the little finger under the palm is another way to check the span.

- As you release, shake hands with the target arrow (Figure 2.16A and 2.16B).
- Visualize gripping a suitcase handle with your thumb to the left (left handers, thumb is to the right). Now on your swing and delivery, keep the thumb and fingers in that same position and do not let the suitcase go broadside to the target at any point in the swing (Figure 2.17).
- Observe your wrist when holding the ball. It should be straight without any wrinkles on the inside or outside of it (Figure 2.18).

Figure 2.16A
Right Handers—You can attain the proper hand position by visualizing that you are shaking hands with the target.

Figure 2.16B
Left Handers—You can attain the proper hand position by visualizing that you are shaking hands with the target.

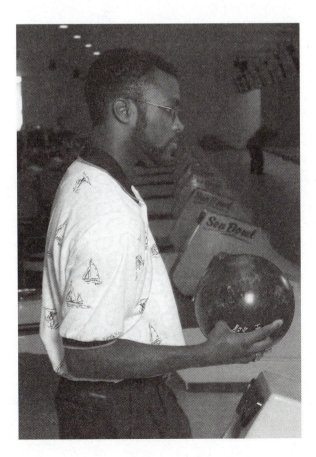

Figure 2.18
In the stance and swing, a straight wrist should be maintained.

Figure 2.17
The thumb should be facing toward the body during the swing.

3

Stance, Approach, and Delivery Concepts

Since most of the errors in bowling are directly related to the approach, it is imperative that a basic approach model be developed which utilizes concepts applicable to everyone. Of the millions of bowlers in the world, no two bowlers bowl exactly the same. This is due to many variables, such as the difference in personalities, body structure, strength, and motivation. Sometimes it is very difficult to distinguish between a person's style and those principles and concepts that are common to all good bowlers.

There are at least four fundamental concepts that apply to all bowlers—good flexibility, balance, timing, and direction. All bowlers need to incorporate these concepts into their game through the practice of efficient movement principles. In this developmental process, the goal should be the fluid integration of the mechanical principles while acquiring a natural feeling for the rhythm of the approach and delivery.

Flexibility and Stance

Once the point of origin for the approach has been established, it is important that the body assume a flexible position before starting the approach. This flexibility in the beginning will follow the bowler throughout the entire delivery and, once lost, cannot be retrieved.

Flexibility is ensured by making several conscious body adjustments in the stance position. **For right handers** to prepare for a four-step approach, the bowler

Figure 3.1A
Right hander—The placement of the toe of the right foot opposite the instep of the left foot.

Figure 3.1B
Left hander—The placement of the toe of the left foot opposite the instep of the right foot.

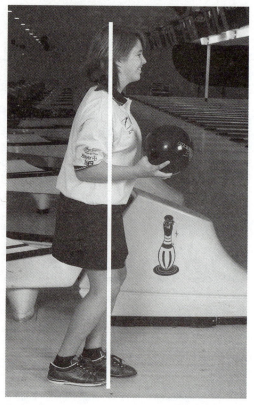

Figure 3.2
The vertical balance line in the stance.

should place the left foot slightly forward of the right so the toe of the right foot is somewhere near the instep of the left foot. The feet are parallel, and about two inches apart (Figure 3.1A). The mass of the body weight should be shifted to the ball of the left foot. These two actions will result in a bowler automatically stepping out with the right foot, eliminating the worry of which foot steps first. **For left handers** to prepare for a four-step approach, the bowler should place the right foot slightly forward of the left so the toe of the left foot is somewhere near the instep of the

right foot. The feet are parallel, and about two inches apart (Figure 3.1B). The mass of the body weight should be shifted to the ball of the right foot. These two actions will result in a bowler automatically stepping out with the left foot, eliminating the worry of which foot steps forward first.

The most important ingredient in our flexibility concept is the establishment of a small degree of flexion in the knees. It is this knee flexion that allows all other things to happen correctly. To maintain good body balance, the bowler should lean forward slightly from the hips, keeping the back relatively straight.

Balance and the Stance

Good balance is a very important aspect of bowling. The **vertical balance line** can be found in an upright body simply by drawing an imaginary straight line from the shoulders through the knees perpendicular to the floor. The more the knees bend, the more the shoulders have to tilt forward in order for the body to remain in balance. When a bowler is balanced, he or she will feel comfortable (Figure 3.2).

Figure 3.3
Right Hander—Holding the ball off the right side of the body.

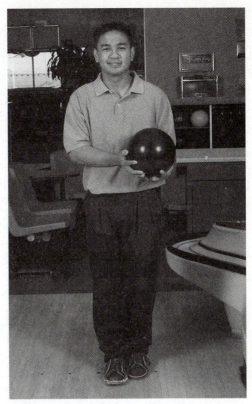

Figure 3.4
Left Hander—Holding the ball off to the left side of the body.

The ball should be supported in the non-bowling hand until the point of origin on the approach is reached. When ready to assume the stance position, insert the fingers into the ball, followed by the thumb. The thumb should be inserted all the way to the webbing. Then, roll the ball from the non-bowling hand to the bowling hand. **Right handers** will have the thumb and fingers at the 10 and 4 o'clock position. It is recommended that the right-handed bowler hold the ball toward the right side of the body, approximately at waist level with the right forearm resting on the hip (Figure 3.3). **Left handers** should insert their thumb and fingers at 2 and 8 o'clock position and hold the ball to the left side of the body, approximately at waist level with the left forearm resting on the hip (Figure 3.4).

Many problems will stem from a ball held in the center of the body, primarily because the ball must be swung out and around to clear the hips. This would result in an inconsistent round-house swing, a swing that goes out and away from the body. Since it is important to keep everything in a straight line, holding the ball to the right locates it properly for the pendular swing pattern.

If the ball does not feel comfortable at waist height, it may be adjusted anywhere between the waist and shoulder as long as it remains slightly to the side of the body (Figures 3.3 and 3.4). If held at shoulder height, the elbows would be resting on the hips (Figure 3.5). In this position, the ball is found near the balance line regardless of whether it is waist or shoulder high. When balanced, the ball will not feel as heavy as it would if held in front of the bowler outside the balance line. Again, it should feel comfortable. We are well on the way to a good approach when we have established a balanced stance position with a degree of flexibility (Figure 3.6).

Timing and Pushaway

The most important part of the bowling approach is the pushaway. It creates timing for the entire approach, swing, and delivery. The **pushaway** is the movement of the ball away from the body which sets the approach and the swing in motion.

The key feature of this concept is that the ball initiates all movement. The ball is moved approximately 3 inches outward and downward to a point where the elbow straightens. The left hand leaves the ball at the end of the pushaway movement. At this point, the balance line of the stance has been intentionally destroyed. Since an unbalanced position has been assumed, the bowler will tilt further forward and react by taking a step in order to keep the body from falling forward (Figures 3.7 and 3.8). This cause-and-effect motion will always happen at the same identical point, consistently and automatically.

The length of the first step is in direct relationship to the length of the pushaway. The farther out the ball is pushed, the longer the first step will be. It is recommended that the first step be fairly short in order to maintain a forward flex of the body. If the pushaway goes up and out, it will force a longer first step, causing the body to lean backward, resulting in the loss of good vertical line and flexibility.

To check for proper timing of the swing in relation to the steps, the second step should be observed. On the second step, the ball should be straight down in the swing (Figure 3.9).

Remember: Move the ball out and in a downward direction and let the feet follow the natural urge to put the body into motion.

Self Evaluation Questions

1. What are the ingredients of a good stance?

2. How can flexibility be introduced into the stance?

Figure 3.5
The ball at shoulder level in the stance.

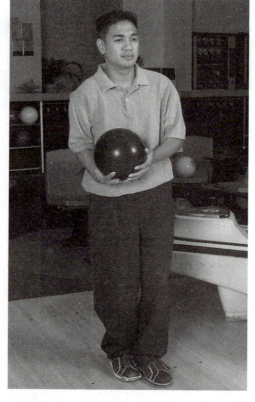

Figure 3.6
In the stance, the bowler should maintain a balanced and flexible position.

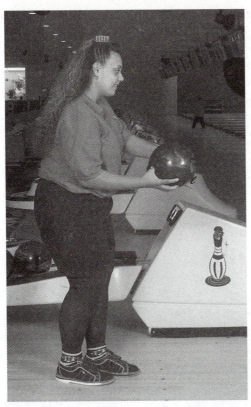

Figure 3.7
The pushaway initiates all movement in the approach.

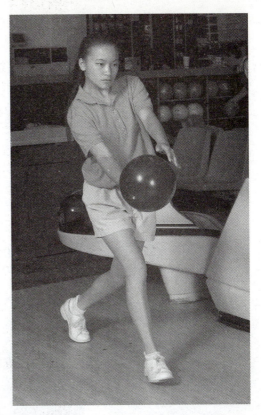

Figure 3.8
The downward direction of the pushaway showing the straightening of the elbow.

Figure 3.9
The point to best check for proper swing and foot coordination is on the second step. The ball should be in the downward position.

Flexibility and Balance in the Approach

The flexibility and balance obtained in the stance should follow

throughout the entire approach. In order to maintain the **vertical balance line** in the approach, flex the knees and take shuffling steps on the balls of the feet instead of using walking steps with a heel-toe action. A **shuffle** is merely a graceful gliding or skating motion across the surface of the approach. This gliding action prevents the body from bouncing up and down

and breaking the rhythm of the approach and swing.

The four-step approach is really three shuffles and a slide. With each shuffle the knees progressively increase their flexion, allowing the body and the ball to be progressively lowered toward the floor for a smooth delivery (Figure 3.10).

a

b

c

d

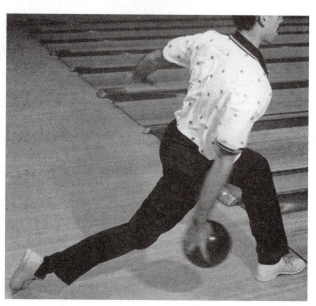

e

Figure 3.10
Showing the increased knee flexion during the entire approach.

Direction in the Approach and Delivery

The last concept in the approach model is **direction.** This concept includes achieving direction toward the target, accuracy in terms of the release, a complete follow-through, and the finishing position.

A good swing will have the following ingredients resulting in the needed accuracy:

● The ball should swing through a natural pendular arc at its own rate of speed. The speed of the swing is directly related to the

length of the arm and the weight of the ball.
● The height of the arc in the backswing should equal the height of the pushaway.
● The arm should follow the natural swing of the ball. The bowler adjusts the rate of the steps to the swing rather than intentionally tampering with the pendular swing in order to match the feet.
● The pendular swing should remain in a straight line with the elbow "grazing" the hip as it moves back and forth.
● On the downswing going into the release, a slight acceleration often occurs providing extra impetus to the "lift" and rotation mechanism at the point of release.

The Release

Right handers: For the beginning bowler the release is very simple. The 10–4 o'clock position (2–8 o'clock for left handers) that was established in the stance is maintained throughout the swing and is still present in the finishing position (Figure 3.11).

The wrist remains firm and straight and the forearm rotates minimally in the swing and release. The sliding foot should point toward the target (Figure 3.12A).

As the ball is released on the far side of the foul line, the thumb should come out of the ball before

Figure 3.11

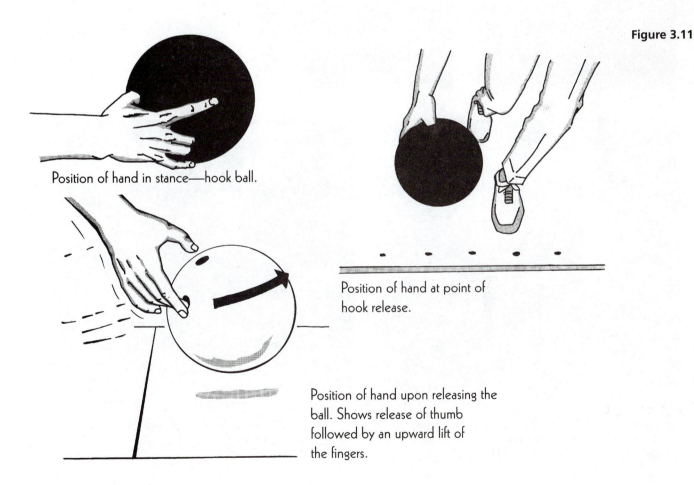

Position of hand in stance—hook ball.

Position of hand at point of hook release.

Position of hand upon releasing the ball. Shows release of thumb followed by an upward lift of the fingers.

the fingers, allowing the lifting action of the fingers in the 4 o'clock position to occur as the ball starts upward in the pendular swing (Figures 3.13 and 3.14). This creates a force off the center of the ball that results in a right-to-left rotation of the ball. The resultant ball roll will find the ball going straight approximately two-thirds of the way down the lane and then, due to the frictional forces equalizing, the ball will start hooking from right to left (left handers, from left to right). This action allows the ball to be rolled over the second arrow (10th board) and hook into the 1–3 pocket (1–2 pocket for left handers) (17th board) at the proper angle (Figure 3.15).

Left handers: For the beginning left-handed bowler, the release is very simple. The 2–8 o'clock position that was established in the stance is maintained throughout the swing and is still present in the finishing position. The wrist remains firm and straight and the forearm rotates minimally in the swing and release. The sliding foot should point toward the target (Figure 3.12B). As the ball is released on the far side of the foul line, the thumb should come out of the ball before the fingers, allowing the lifting action of the fingers in the

8 o'clock position to occur as the ball starts upward in the pendular swing (Figures 3.13 and 3.14). This creates a force off the center of the ball which results in a left-to-right rotation of the ball. The resultant ball roll will find the ball going straight approximately two-thirds of the way down the lane and then, due to the frictional forces equalizing, the ball will start hooking from the left to the right. This action allows the ball to be rolled over the second arrow (10th board from the left) and hooking into the 1–2 pocket (17th board) at the proper angle.

Self Evaluation Questions

1. What initiates the forward motion of the body?

2. Where is the ball moved in the pushaway phase?

3. With each shuffle, what happens to the knees?

4. In what position are the thumb and fingers held throughout the swing and delivery?

5. What happens at the delivery with the thumb? The fingers?

6. On which target arrow should the ball roll?

Figure 3.12A
The 10–4 o'clock position should be held throughout the swing and delivery; the wrist remains firm and straight, and sliding foot points towards target.

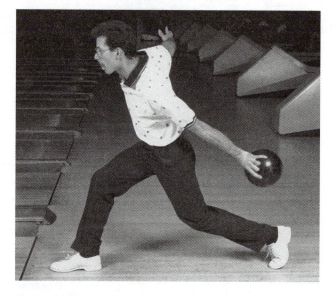

Figure 3.12B
For a left-handed bowler, the 2–8 o'clock position should be held throughout the swing and delivery.

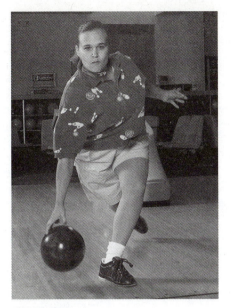

Figure 3.13
The thumb exits the ball before the fingers release the ball.

Figure 3.14
The "lift" placed on the ball as it is released while the arm continues upward into the follow-through.

Figure 3.15
The follow-through.

The Follow-Through

The last factor that assists in achieving good direction is the **extension or follow-through.** A good extension (follow-through) will find the bowler's eyes still focusing on the target and the straightened bowling arm moving forward in direct line with the target arrow (Figure 3.15).

Vertical Balance Line and the Delivery

Throughout the stance and the approach, the shoulders are kept over flexed knees for the maintenance of good balance. This already established **vertical**

balance line is also very important in a bowler's finishing position to allow a smooth and consistent delivery. By bending the knees rather than bending at the waist or dropping the shoulders, the bowler can get closer to the floor, which aids in placing the ball on the lane rather than dropping it (Figure 3.16). After a well-balanced delivery, the body can maintain a comfortable follow-through position (Figure 3.17).

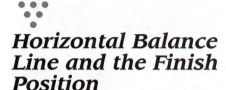

Horizontal Balance Line and the Finish Position

Besides the vertical balance line, there is also a proper **horizontal balance line** that is critical in the finish position. In order to counterbalance the weight of the bowling ball that is moving in front and to the side of the body, the body must make other adjustments. The opposite arm becomes a counterbalance by being stretched

out and angles a little backwards. This procedure assists in keeping the shoulders and hips square to the target.

Right handers: The most crucial adjustment for horizontal balance at the delivery is accomplished for right-handed bowlers by stretching the right leg backwards in a straightened position and letting it drift to the left in a pigeon-toed position. By turning the toe inward in this pigeon-toed position, the hip curls under, opening the right side (Figure 3.18A). This allows the ball to swing in an unobstructed straight line toward the target. Caution should be taken here because if the leg is kicked around behind, it will jerk the torso out of alignment. To prevent this from happening, the bowler should try to keep the toe on the approach and let it slide into place.

Left handers: The most crucial adjustment for horizontal balance at the delivery for a left hander is accomplished by stretching the left

leg backwards in a straightened position and letting it drift to the right in a pigeon-toed position. By turning the toe inward in this pigeon-toed position, the hip curls under, opening the left side (Figure 3.18B). This allows the ball to swing in an unobstructed straight line toward the target. Caution should be taken here because if the leg is kicked around behind, it will jerk the torso out of alignment. To prevent this from happening, the bowler should try to keep the toe on the approach and let it slide into place.

Hand and Arm Position in the Follow-through

After the ball has been delivered, the bowling arm continues to move forward in a direct line with the target arrow. The finish position should find a ninety-degree angle

Figure 3.16
Increased knee flexion lowers the body to the necessary delivery level.

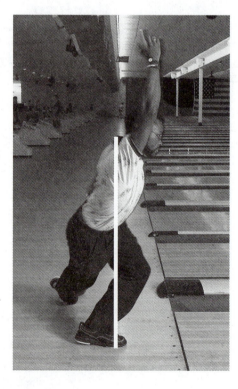

Figure 3.17
The vertical balance line is maintained throughout the delivery and follow-through.

Figure 3.18A, B
Counterbalancing the weight of the ball by extending the opposite arm (horizontal balance).

a

b

formed between the shoulder, the arm, and the target with the fingers curled into the palm of the hand. The eyes remain focused on the target arrow and should be able to identify the exact board over which the ball is rolled.

Self Evaluation Questions

1. How is the body lowered in order to lay the ball on the floor in the delivery?

2. What body adjustment must be made to counterbalance the weight of the ball in the approach? The delivery?

3. Explain the action of the trailing leg in the delivery.

4. Explain the finish position of the arms and fingers.

Summary of Bowling Fundamentals for Right-handed Bowlers (Figures 3.19 and 3.20)

Stance

● The left foot is placed slightly forward of the right with the majority of the body weight on the ball of the left foot.

● The knees are unlocked and slightly flexed. The shoulders are tilted forward slightly from the hips and should be directly above the knees.

● The ball is supported in the non-bowling hand until the point of origin is found and the stance has been assumed.

● The thumb and fingers of the bowling hand are now inserted into the ball (fingers first) at the 10 and 4 o'clock position. Then it

is rolled from the non-bowling hand to the bowling hand.

● The ball is held to the right front of the body at approximately waist height with the forearm resting on the hip. The ball is near the vertical balance line drawing a line through the shoulders and knees and is supported slightly by the non-bowling hand.

● The shoulders and hips should be square to the intended line of ball roll.

Pushaway

● The most crucial part of the approach and swing is in timing the pushaway with the approach.

● The pushaway is a movement of the ball out from the body in a downward direction resulting in the straightening of the bowling arm.

● The pushaway action puts the body in an unbalanced position and will cause the body to take a step forward.

● The step forward will be with the right foot, which was the unweighted back foot in the stance.

Figure 3.19
A side angle view of a four-step approach.

a

b

c

d

e

f

Approach
- During the approach, the feet will take three shuffle steps and a slide.
- Each shuffle step will find the knees progressively more flexed.
- The shuffle should be in a straight line moving toward the target arrow.
- The eyes of the bowler are focused solely on the target.
- If the swing and the approach are coordinated, the ball will be just starting to move upward into the backswing on the second step.

Swing
- The weight of the ball straightens the elbow on the pushaway that is the start of the arc for the pendular swing.
- The ball swings straight back in the natural pendular swing to the height of the backswing, somewhere between the waist and the shoulder.
- During this swing the 10–4 o'clock thumb-finger position is maintained with a straight elbow and firm wrist.
- The wrist remains firm through the swing, including the peak backswing position.

- The shoulders and hips are square to the target throughout the swing.
- The non-bowling arm is extended to the side and slightly back for balance.

Delivery
- The slide is accomplished by bending the knees to the point where the ball can swing out on the lane without being dropped or dropping the shoulder.
- The shoulders are moved forward from the hips and aligned directly over the knees in order to keep the vertical balance line intact.

a

b

c

d

e

f

g

Figure 3.20
Front view of a four-step approach.

- In order to counterbalance the weight of the ball that has moved in front of the vertical balance line, the right leg is extended back and drifts to the left in a pigeon-toed fashion.
- The hips and shoulders remain square to the target.
- The ball is released on the far side of the foul line as it starts upward in the pendular swing.
- On the release, the thumb and fingers are still in the 10–4 o'clock position.
- The thumb is automatically released from the ball first and then the fingers are released with an upward lifting action. The off-center lift will cause the ball to have a right-to-left (counter-clockwise) rotation, resulting in a slight hook.

Follow-through
- The eyes remain focused on the target arrow.
- The bowling arm moves forward in a direct line with the target arrow.
- The fingers are curled toward the palm of the hand.
- The finish position is a ninety-degree angle formed between the shoulder, the arm, and the target.

Summary of Bowling Fundamentals for Left-handed Bowlers (Figure 3.21)

Stance
- The right foot is placed forward of the left with the majority of the body weight on the ball of the right foot.

Figure 3.21
A side angle view of a left-handed four-step approach.

- The knees are unlocked and slightly flexed. The shoulders are tilted forward slightly from the hips and should be directly over the knees.
- The ball is supported in the right hand while taking your position at your point of origin.
- The thumb and fingers of the bowling hand are now inserted into the ball at the 2 and 8 o'clock position, fingers first. Then the ball is rolled from the non-bowling hand to the bowling hand.
- The ball is held to the left front of the body at approximately waist height with the forearm resting on the hip. The ball is near the vertical balance line drawing a line through the shoulders and knees and is supported slightly by the non-bowling hand.
- The shoulders and hips should be square to the intended line of the ball roll.

Pushaway
- The crucial part of the approach and swing is in timing the pushaway with the approach.
- The pushaway is a movement of the ball out from the body in a downward direction resulting in the straightening of the bowling arm.
- The pushaway action puts the body in an unbalanced position and will cause the body to take a step forward.
- The step forward will be with the left foot which was the unweighted back foot in the stance.

Approach
- During the approach, the feet will take three shuffle steps and a slide.
- Each shuffle step finds the knees progressively more flexed.

- The shuffle should be in a straight line moving toward the target arrow.
- The eyes of the bowler are focused solely on the target.
- If the swing and the approach are coordinated, the ball will be just starting to move upward into the backswing on the second step.

Swing
- The weight of the ball straightens the elbow on the pushaway, which is the start of the arc for the pendular swing.
- The ball swings straight back in the natural pendular swing to the height of the backswing, somewhere between the waist and shoulders.
- During this swing, the 2–8 o'clock thumb–finger position is maintained with a straight elbow and firm wrist.
- The wrist remains firm throughout the swing, including the peak backswing position.
- The non-bowling arm (right) is extended to the side and slightly back for balance.

Delivery
- The slide is accomplished by bending the knee to the point where the ball can swing out on the lane without being dropped or dropping the shoulder.
- The shoulders are moved forward from the hips and aligned directly over the knees in order to keep the vertical line intact.
- In order to counterbalance the weight of the ball that has moved in front of the vertical balance line, the left leg is extended back and drifts to the right in a pigeon-toed fashion.
- The hips and shoulders remain square to the target.
- The ball is released on the far side of the foul line as it starts upward in the pendular swing.

- On the release, the thumb and fingers are still in the 2–8 o'clock position.
- The thumb is automatically released from the ball first and then the fingers are released with an upward lifting action. The off-center lift will cause the ball to have a left-to-right (clockwise) rotation, resulting in a slight hook.

Follow-through
- The eyes remain focused on the target arrow until the ball passes over the target.
- The bowling arm moves forward in a direct line with the target arrow.
- The fingers are curled toward the palm of the hand.
- The finish position is a ninety-degree angle formed between the shoulder, the arm, and the target.

Hints for Success

Approach
- To practice shuffling without the ball, try keeping your footwork quiet and noiseless. The noise should resemble sandpaper rubbing across wood.
- To increase the shuffling action, visualize "sneaking up" to the foul line.
- To maintain balance and to keep your body from bouncing during the approach, visualize approaching the line with a glass of water on each shoulder.
- To keep yourself from "drifting," visualize taking the approach on a balance beam.

Arm Swing
- To emphasize the natural pendular motion of the arm

swing, visualize the arm as a pendulum on a large clock. Then take practice swings, allowing the ball to swing in a natural pendular motion and rate of speed.

● To assist in keeping the swing straight, try to feel your elbow grazing past the hip.

Ball Release

● To assist in getting more "lift," visualize squeezing a gun trigger as the ball comes off the hand in the release.

● To assist in getting more lift, feel the finger pressure in the ball and, upon release, curl the fingers into the palm of your hand.

Body Balance in the Release and Follow-through

● To assist in staying low and in balance throughout the release and follow-through, visualize extending the knee cap (not the head) over the foul line while keeping the slide foot flat on the approach.

● To ensure the proper use of the balance arm and avoid a "dropped shoulder," visualize holding a bucket of water with the left hand (left handers—right hand).

Follow-through

● To ensure a complete follow-through and correct direction, visualize holding a glass of water in the bowling hand and tossing the water up and over your shoulder, keeping the elbow straight as long as possible.

● To maintain the follow-through and body stability at the foul line, "stay still" until the ball passes the target arrow.

4

Principles of Movement Applied to Bowling

As was previously noted, it is important to know the "whys and wherefores" when learning or trying to improve a skill. By knowing the concepts and principles involved in effective movement, learning can be enhanced by making it more meaningful. Analysis and error correction then becomes second nature.

We are most likely all familiar with Newton's Law of Motion that states, "An object which is at rest or is in motion will remain at rest or in motion at the same speed, in a straight line, unless acted upon by an outside force." This principle will be our chief guide throughout our bowling swing, approach, and delivery. In order to analyze each phase of this physical law, many other concepts and principles enter the picture.

Weight of the Ball

It has been previously noted that weight is an important consideration when selecting a ball. Each bowler should select a ball that is as heavy as he or she can control. The reason for this is quite obvious when one considers the principles of force and gravity. In an underarm swing pattern, gravity will cause the ball to swing in a straight, pendular fashion unless restricted or acted upon by another force. If the ball is heavy enough, and if a bowler will allow this natural swing, force will be produced by gravity and momentum, not by the bowler "muscling" and forcing the ball. In this natural swing pattern, the direction of the swing will always remain constant and, if lined up correctly, will remain in a straight line. If the ball is too light, a bowler has the tendency to push or pull the ball off his or her natural swing line, resulting in inconsistency. Additionally, a heavier ball will usually result in greater pin fall. This is because a heavier ball does not deflect as easily as a lighter ball when it contacts the weight of the pins.

Force Production

It is essential that enough force be generated at delivery to allow the ball to travel effectively on course. Force is generated during the swing and the approach.

Swing

The production of gravitational force in the swing is directly related to the following principle: *The greater distance the swinging object travels, the more time for gravity to act on the ball, thereby producing more force.* Consequently, a ball held higher in the stance, all things being equal, would result in a longer arc because the backswing would equal the height of the pushaway (Figure 4.1). The ball would be traveling a greater distance, allowing gravity to have more time to act on the ball, resulting in more ball velocity at the time of delivery.

A bowler having trouble producing enough force at the delivery may want to try holding the ball higher in the stance. Gradual changes are recommended to maintain good form and consistency.

Another way of allowing the ball to travel a greater distance in the swing is to lengthen the lever that is moving through space. That lever, the bowler's arm, should be completely straightened in the pushaway and the backswing to allow for maximum length.

Because of the added weight of the ball and the momentum that the ball is gathering, the body must remain stable and firm throughout the entire swing. By stabilizing the shoulder and wrist of the swinging arm, the pendular swing will stay in a straight line. This stabilizing action will also keep the shoulder from dropping and free it from muscle strain. Stabilizing the wrist during all phases of the swing, particularly the backswing, merely keeps the ball from straying off the desired pendular path.

Approach

The main purpose of an approach is to gather the forward body momentum that will be transferred to the ball at the release. Since a gravitational swing alone will not build up enough momentum to roll the ball at a speed great enough to hold the desired line and successfully knock down the pins, it is necessary to add an approach to assist in this force production.

The principle of time and distance becomes important when developing momentum in the approach. The greater the time and

Figure 4.1
The ball can be held high in the stance for the production of more momentum.

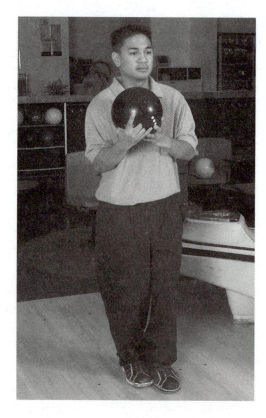

distance over which momentum is developed, the greater the force imparted. Therefore, the longer and faster the approach, all things being equal, the greater the momentum build-up. Many times this results in bowlers running to the foul line from the end of the approach so the ball will have greater momentum. Erroneously, they assume that this fast ball will scare the pins down. Remember, in bowling everything is controlled and coordinated. An approach should only be as long and as fast as needed to coordinate with the swing, to hold the desired line to the pins, and to knock the pins down.

Here are some factors to keep in mind while developing momentum in the approach:

● Shuffle steps will allow for a smoother approach. By keeping the body free from bounding, all energies will be directed to building forward momentum. Outside forces acting on the ball swing will be kept to a minimum and the ball will remain in its natural arc.

● The vertical balance line should be shifted forward throughout the approach. The forward shift of body weight should be from the ankles. This helps in many ways:

1. It will place the center of gravity in front of the pushing foot for ease in building momentum during the steps.
2. It will assure a smooth approach by allowing the knees to act as shock absorbers in each step.
3. It will increase the arc of the ball due to the body leaning slightly forward, allowing for greater force production.
4. It assures the body a position over a bent knee upon release for a smooth, straight delivery.
5. It forces the point of maximum momentum to coincide with the ball delivery over the foul line.
6. It allows the arm swing to continue forward for a greater distance in the follow through for maximum momentum and direction.

It is almost impossible for a bowler who is standing erect or approaching in an erect fashion to shift his or her weight forward upon the delivery of the ball. In this erect position, the body's center of gravity is high and the body's weight is slightly back. As a result, the ball will be released beside or behind the left foot, with the swing going in an upward direction and the ball crossing the lane (Figure 4.2).

If the forward weight shift comes from the waist rather than the ankles, the hips will remain high, resulting in an unbalanced body during approach and delivery, with the majority of the force production going downward into the floor rather than out onto the lane. The resultant follow-through will be incomplete with very little chance for "lift" to be placed on the ball (Figure 4.3).

● At all times during the approach, the toes, feet, and body should be going in a straight line for maximum mechanical efficiency. This allows the feet to push directly from behind and also allows for all momentum to be directed and released in the direction of the target.

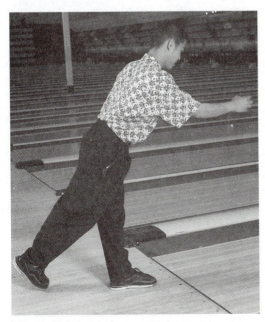

Figure 4.2
Releasing the ball with little knee bend usually results in a loss of accuracy.

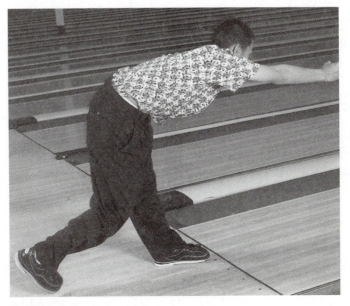

Figure 4.3
Bending from the waist results in a loss of power at the release point.

How much momentum or **ball speed** is really needed to get an effective ball roll? It should be noted that all good bowlers develop a specific optimal ball speed. Research has determined the optimal average ball speed to be delivered at 17 miles per hour, or 2.4 seconds from the point of release to the head pin. At this speed, all governing forces will be in proper balance, allowing the ball to hit pins with the most effective impact. This speed allows the pins to topple in a domino fashion rather than flying upward as with a fast ball. A slower ball will deflect as it hits the pins causing ineffective pin action.

Hook Ball and Momentum

When first released, the ball is traveling at its maximum speed, and slides more than rolls in a straight line. This is partly due to the speed of the ball on the lane. Frictional forces build up between the ball and the lane and slow the ball. As the ball slows, the side rotation imparted by the fingers lifting the ball off the center of gravity (4 o'clock position for right handers and 8 o'clock for left handers) now takes effect. When this side rotation becomes greater than the forward roll, the ball begins to hook toward the pocket.

When the ball speed, forward roll, and side rotation forces are in proper balance, the result will be an effective, consistent, working hook ball.

Straight Ball Principles

Throughout this text, the authors have selected to only teach the rolling of an effective hook ball. It is the ball roll of choice, primarily due to the carrying action at the pins. However, it is foreseen that many beginning bowlers may release the ball as a straight ball with the thumb and fingers at 12 and 6 o'clock, resulting in a ball that goes straight down the lane without any side rotation. This ball roll does possess a lot of consistency and accuracy regardless of lane conditions, but it is less effective when it contacts the pins. This is primarily due to the ball deflecting away from the center pins as it contacts the first in the set. The result: the pins behind the head pin often remain untouched.

Correction Suggestions for Straight Ball

Remember that the thumb and fingers are the problem areas that need correcting at the moment of release. The thumb and fingers are at the 12 and 6 o'clock position instead of the 10 and 4 o'clock position for right handers and the 8 and 2 o'clock position for left handers. The result: a straight ball. Two different things may be causing this finger positioning on the ball. First, the bowler may have placed his or her fingers in that position at the stance and carried it throughout the swing, approach, and delivery. Or, the bowler started with the fingers in the hook ball position and during the backswing rotated the palm of the hand down and flexed the wrist backward (as he or she would do in an underhanded softball throw). The forward swing and release would probably find the fingers remaining in this 12 and 6 o'clock position and pulling up through the middle of the ball from underneath. Again, the result would be a straight ball. It is imperative that the fingers stay in the hook ball position throughout the stance, swing, and release to ensure the rotation on the ball that will result in a hook. (See the Instructor's Manual for drills and the Advanced Section of *Right Down Your Alley*.)

Backup Ball Principles

The backup ball is often referred to as a reverse hook but it is really an offshoot of the full roller or straight ball. It hooks from right to left for right handers (left to right for left handers). It is usually due to the thumb rotating from the 10 o'clock to the 12 o'clock position (right handers) or the 2 o'clock to the 12 o'clock position (left handers). This is an exaggeration of the straight ball release. Many bowlers continue the finger and hand rotation past the 12 o'clock position in the release. The result is a ball that rotates in a clockwise position for right handers and a counter-clockwise rotation for left handers. The ball then has a reverse hooking action. This ball is fairly effective as it contacts the pins due to the ball rotation and "digging" action. However, the big drawback is the lack of consistency in the amount of the reverse hook due to the free rotation of the hand at the release point. It is difficult to release at the same exact point of the hand rotation.

Correction Suggestions for the Backup Ball

The main correction of a backup ball is to somehow ensure that the bowler takes a hook ball finger and hand position at the time of the stance and maintains that hand position without any wrist or forearm rotation throughout the swing, approach, and delivery. At times, there is an overemphasis of the thumb and finger position by placing them at 9 and 3 o'clock (right handers) or 3 and 9 o'clock (left handers). At the release point, the bowler should try to follow-through with the index finger pointing toward the target with the fingernail facing up. This automatically puts the thumb in a 9 o'clock position (right handers) and 3 o'clock (left handers). (Additional suggestions may be found in the Instructor's Manual and in the Advanced Section of *Right Down Your Alley*.)

Correction Suggestions for Changing Ball Speeds

Any time changes are to be made in the speed of the ball, it is of great importance to maintain good coordination, flexibility, balance, and timing of the swing and approach. When a bowler is having trouble generating enough speed on the ball, it will hook too far to the left. This is due to too little slide and too much side rotation. Any of five

different corrections may resolve the problem.

Not Enough Ball Speed
● The ball could be put into the swing a tad earlier to create a more rapid approach tempo.
● The ball may be held higher in the stance, which will automatically create a longer arc.
● The ball may be pushed away a bit farther on the pushaway.
● A 5-step approach may be used to give a longer approach to produce more forward momentum.

If a 5-step approach is used, the ball is held higher and pushed out a little farther in order for the swing to be properly coordinated.

● The approach may be started at least 6 inches further back.
● Think of reducing the overall effort put into the approach by 25 percent.
● A lighter ball could be used.

Some rethinking may be in order for those who are intent on throwing the ball as hard as they can. They are probably leaving pocket splits, often the 5 pin, and not getting effective pin action. These bowlers will continue to do so unless their mental attitude is changed by someone who can prove why that type of ball is not the most effective. A fast ball results in too much slide and not enough side rotation so the hook is very minimal. The following suggestions could be used.

Too Much Ball Speed
● In the stance, hold the ball lower to decrease the resistance of the swing.
● The pushaway could be shortened or de-emphasized.
● The knees can be flexed more because it is very difficult for anyone to move fast with flexed knees.

● Use the force of gravity to move the ball in the swing rather than forcing the ball. Flex the knees more, pushing the ball out lower, and not quite so far. This should allow the bowler to feel the natural weight of the ball swinging his or her arm rather than his or her arm doing the swinging. He or she should constantly feel relaxed.
● The approach could be started at least 6 inches closer.
● Think of reducing the overall effort put into the approach by 25 percent.
● A heavier ball could be used.

Accuracy and Consistency Principles

Once force production is present, a bowler must move his or her force in a consistent movement pattern in order to ensure accuracy. To establish accuracy and consistency in the swing, approach, and delivery, everything must move in straight lines toward the designated target.

The swing must stay in a straight forward and backward arc. Holding the ball off to the right side while in the stance will assure that it will travel in this straight line instead of moving in a circular pattern around the hips. Stabilizing the shoulders and wrist in the swing will also assist in keeping the swing straight.

The approach must be in a fairly straight line while moving toward the designated target. The shoulders and hips should be perpendicular to this target line as the feet move in a straight line toward the target. By keeping the upper body position

Figure 4.4
Upon delivery, the entire body is square to the target.

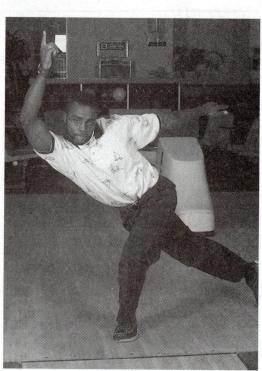

Figure 4.5
Keeping the shoulders and hips square to the target results in more accuracy.

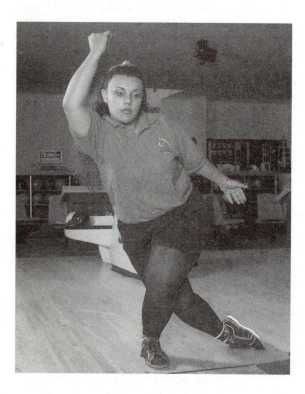

square to the target, the swing will also stay square to the target (Figure 4.4).

The 10 o'clock thumb position for right handers and 2 o'clock for left handers must remain constant throughout the swing. In order to maintain this position, the wrist must remain firm and the forearm must not rotate.

Upon the release of the ball, everything is still square to the intended line of aim: the shoulders, the hips, the swing, and the follow-through. In order to fulfill and control the square-to-square concept, the entire body must be in perfect balance (Figure 4.5).

Controlling the entire body in the approach and the swing will ensure the bowler of rolling the ball the same way time after time. Once this consistency is conquered, the bowler can now start making accurate adjustments.

In summary, looking back upon Newton's Law of Motion, which states an object which is at rest or in motion will remain at rest or in motion at the same speed, in a straight line, unless acted upon by an outside force, we find that every part of this law applies to bowling force production and accuracy. It is every bowler's object to control the

variables in the skill of bowling in order to reach his or her potential. Once these variables are identified, error correction is also very easy.

References

Broer, Marion R. 1966. *Efficiency of human movement.* 2nd ed. Philadelphia: Saunders.

Culver, Elizabeth J. 1964. "Bowling." In Ainsworth, Dorothy S.: *Individual sports for women*, 4th ed. Philadelphia: Saunders.

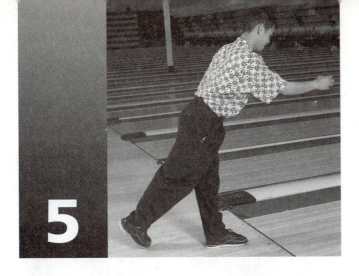

5

Common Errors and Corrective Actions

The following chart of common bowling errors, effects, and corrective actions will assist a bowler or an instructor in developing diagnostic skills. However, due to the great number of movement variables and the interrelationship of these movements, it is impossible to cover every possible error and give the correct diagnosis for that particular individual's error. This chart is intended to assist the instructor in experiencing and sharpening diagnostic skills by analyzing the most common errors found in bowling. The concept of the error and corrections can more easily be identified by the cause-and-effect relationship as stated in the charts.

ERROR	CAUSE	EFFECT	CORRECTION
General:			
Lack of pin action	Lack of lift Lack of hook Lack of ball revolutions Ball rolls over thumb hole Lofting ball Overreaching Ball too light Late release Thumb hole too tight Improper pitches Ball line too far inside Ball line too far outside Skidding ball	Pins are left standing	Note: Check all corrections for these causes. Angle and proper revolutions are key to good pin action.
Backup ball (reverse hook)	Lack of knowledge of ball release and types of roll Thumb position at 12 o'clock and hand rotation Fingers in 6–7 o'clock position Starting with straight ball when learning to bowl Flexed wrist in stance or release Holding the ball in the middle of one's body Dropping right shoulder	Maximum ball deflection Lack of lift due to hyperextended wrist rotation Lack of consistency	Correct starting position (lining up shoulder with arrow). Hold ball in 8 or 9 o'clock position in stance. Firm wrist by pressing down with two outside fingers. Hold ball with forearm resting on hip in stance. Flex knees.
Stance:			
Feet too far apart	Attempt at body balance	Drifting Waddling	Move feet closer together.
Improper distribution of weight	Attempt at body balance	Not starting automatically with proper foot	Place most of the weight on balance-side foot.
Stiff knees	Bending too much at waist or leaning too far back	Large, awkward steps or not shuffling	Flex both knees equally.
Excessive forward body angle	Bending too much at waist	Stiff knees Loss of balance Tendency to rush	Straighten body enough to restore correct balance line.
Ball held too high	Ball held too high trying to get speed Slight aiming over ball	Release balance hand too soon Pushaway too long Steps too long Excessive approach speed High backswing	Establish ball height which will give smooth, controlled pendulum swing and desired speed.
Ball held too low	Excessive bending at waist	Push directly away too much Carrying ball during first step Timing off—body ahead of ball disrupts pendulum swing	Raise ball to desired height.
One heel up	One stiff knee	Balance and weight overshifted	Flex both knees equally.

ERROR	CAUSE	EFFECT	CORRECTION
Ball held in center of body	Ball feels comfortable equally supported with both hands	Tendency to hold thumb at 12 o'clock Tendency to flex wrist Tendency to develop outside-in arm swing or wrap-around swing Tendency to develop drift to left	Move ball position in line with right shoulders.
Elbow not tucked in	Elbow not tucked in to hip in stance Holding ball in center of body	Outside-in or wrap around swing Incorrect and changing thumb position in swing	Place forearm on hip bone.
Wrist bent (Gooseneck)	Not enough pressure with index and little finger Loose grip Incorrect span	Ball slides too much and deflects Inconsistent delivery Painful knuckles	Press firmly against ball with two outside fingers or give support to wrist.
Wrist cupped	Overly firm wrist muscle flex	Locked elbow and shoulder, prohibiting natural pendulum swing and release Inconsistent delivery Restricted backswing	Relax arm and let ball drop naturally. Feel ball weight on fingers in stance.
Improper spread of outside fingers	Outside fingers either spread or close to middle fingers Lack of understanding of the effects of spread of either or both index or little finger	Not achieving maximum hooking/hitting potential	Hold outside fingers close if little or no turn desired. Spread index finger for semi-roller, if extra turn desired. Spread little finger for full-roller, if extra turn desired.
Weak grip	Not enough pressure exerted with two middle fingers	Too much fluctuation of hand during swing Dropped ball	Put tension in wrist and fingers.
	Not enough pressure with two outside fingers Short span and/or large holes	Lack of backswing No lift	Select ball with proper span and hole sizes.
Lack of concentration	Lack of confidence Distraction on approach Wandering mind Eyes not focused on target Self-induced pressure	Imperfect execution of delivery Carry-over frustration Low scores Inconsistent approach method	Develop simple, relaxed concentration—not grim, lip-biting, teeth-gritting determination.
Lack of relaxation	Grim determination Giving in to pressure of occasion Gripping ball too tightly Lack of proper breathing	Ball steered, pushed, or pulled in delivery Inability to sustain string of strikes	Take a deep breath—exhale. Flex knees. Loosen grip slightly. Feel looseness in elbow. Lean forward slightly, ready for smooth pushaway step.

ERROR	CAUSE	EFFECT	CORRECTION
Pushaway (First Step):			
Ball pushed too high	Attempt to develop speed Ball pushed up more than out Weight is back Ball is too light	Abrupt lowering of ball Low or high backswing Jerky swing Dropped shoulder Poor timing—bowler ahead of ball	Push ball in a downward direction.
Ball lowered too soon (little or no pushaway)	Ball pushed down more than out Attempt to get ball in backswing, quickly Leaning forward in stance Ball too heavy	Muscling the swing Ball not in the appropriate position at conclusion of first step Poor timing—ball is ahead of bowler	Push ball in a downward direction. Check ball weight. Push ball in outward direction. Extend elbows during pushaway.
Pushaway too long	Attempt to straighten arm and extend to full length for full pendulum swing	Step too long Feeling of rushing	Push ball a moderate distance forward and downward. Delay straightening of elbow. Avoid leaning forward with pushaway.
Ball pushed too far right or left	Try to clear the hip Lack of kinesthetic awareness	Developing inside-out or outside-in swing Missing target Dropping shoulder	Hold ball to side of body in front of shoulder and push ball toward target. Maintain thumb position created in stance.
Downswing (Second Step):			
Balance hand released too late	Not taking balance hand off ball Fear of dropping ball	Carrying ball Hurried downswing Stiff approach	The balance hand should be disengaged, just as the first step is completed.
Left hand released too early (Figure 5.1)	Taking balance hand off ball too early	Muscling Hurried swing Dropped shoulder Timing off	The balance hand should be disengaged, just as the first step is completed

Figure 5.1
Release of left hand too soon in downswing.

ERROR	CAUSE	EFFECT	CORRECTION
Ball carried	Balance hand not disengaged Lack of pushaway Not using force of gravity	Timing off Inconsistent ball speed	Move ball first, let feet follow. Balance hand should be disengaged. Let gravitational force act upon the ball.
Lack of counter balance	Balance arm not allowed to attain counter-balance position	Dropped shoulder	Simultaneously with the downward motion of the ball, extend the balance arm to the side of, and slightly away from, body.

Backswing (Third Step):			
	Ball too light	Shoulder/hip rotation	Increase weight of ball.
Backswing too high (Figure 5.2)	Pushaway too high and too forceful Attempt to get speed by deliberately raising ball in backswing Shoulder and hip allowed to tilt forward and rotate	Possible sideways finish on fourth step Sidearming delivery Too much speed	Control pushaway—let natural pendulum swing develop. Do not add speed in swing by "muscling." Flex knees and avoid bending at the waist.
Backswing too low	Inhibited swing Cupped wrist Muscling Ball too heavy	Muscling Forced release Early turn	Develop free pendulum swing. Push the ball slightly higher in pushaway. Decrease weight of ball.

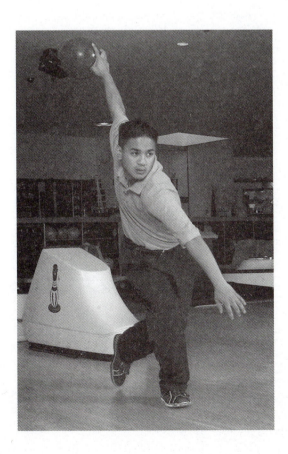

Figure 5.2
Backswing too high.

ERROR	CAUSE	EFFECT	CORRECTION
Backswing (Third Step):			

Shoulder and hip rotation	Pushaway too forceful
	Attempt to get speed by
	  deliberately increasing
	  backswing
		May result in sideways
		  finish in fourth step
		Sidearming delivery
			Control pushaway—
			  develop free pendulum swing.
			Do not add speed to swing
			  by "muscling."
			Maintain consistent thumb
			  position.
			Maintain firm wrist
			  throughout swing.

Hesitation at top of backswing	Bending too far forward Weight on toes Hunching shoulders	Inhibited fluid motion of swing Forced downswing	Restore body balance on balance line. Develop free pendulum swing.

Wrap-around swing	Ball held in center of body
	  in stance
	Ball held to right of
	  shoulders in stance
	Ball pushed to right during
	  first step
		Inconsistent ball path and
		  direction
			Keep shoulders square to
			  target.
			Position ball in line with
			  shoulder and push
			  straight ahead.

Elbow bent	Over-controlling the ball
	Incorrect span
		Inconsistent speed and
		  delivery
		Sidearm release
		Lack of pendular swing
			Extend elbow in pushaway.
			Feel gravitational pull of ball in
			  downswing.

Swing "bumps" outward	Ball pushed away toward left	Misdirected follow-through	Push toward target. Maintain hand and wrist position.

Wrist rotates inward	Shoulders not square to
	  target
		Keep shoulders square to
		  target	

Bowling shoulder dropped	Balance arm too high	Loss of balance to ball side	Maintain balance arm below shoulder level.
Timing (Fourth Step):			

Body ahead of ball	Sliding too far
	Lack of synchronized
	  movement
	Lack of balance line
	Pushaway started late
		Body balance lost
		Hurried released
		Dropped ball
		Pushed or pulled ball
		Sidearming in delivery
			Bring ball forward with
			  slide.
			Restore balance line.
			Slide only as far as body
			  balance can be
			  maintained.
			Move the ball first in
			  pushaway.

Not enough slide	Stance too close to foul line
	Heel-toe approach
	Lack of balance line
	Picking up sliding foot
	Landing heel first
	Lack of flex in sliding knee
		Crowded steps
		Abrupt stop
		Abrupt release
		Difficulty completing
		  follow-through
			Move stance further back.
			Shuffle during delivery.
			Develop balance line.
			Concentrate on sliding last
			  step.
			Keep ball-side foot down
			  longer before raising for
			  balance.

Too much slide	Stance too far from foul
	  line
	Over-emphasis on slide
	Lack of balance line
	Right hip and shoulder
	  remaining back
	Approach too fast
		Too much space for steps
		Right hip and shoulder
		  remaining back
		Improper lift on ball
		Poor balance line
			Move stance closer to foul
			  line.
			Maintain balance line
			  during slide.
			Decrease speed of steps
			  and flex knees.

ERROR	CAUSE	EFFECT	CORRECTION
Sliding on wrong foot (Figure 5.3)	Start approach on wrong foot Timing of steps and swing off	No follow-through off balance Lack of accuracy and consistency	Place most weight on balance-side foot in stance. Practice coordination of steps and swing.
Hop or skip steps	Straightening sliding–side knee, heel comes in contact with approach too soon Ball at top of backswing too soon Poor timing	Erratic release Loss of balance	Restore balance line. Start pushaway later. Extend pushaway further out.
Sliding sideways (Figure 5.4)	Approach too fast Insufficient sliding Lack of knee bend Starting approach too close to foul line Trail leg in open position (not pigeon-toed)	Inconsistent release Dropped ball Improper lift on ball Swinging ball around	Decrease speed of steps and flex knees. Flex sliding knee. Keep trail leg pigeon-toed and in contact with floor.
Off-balance sideways (Figure 5.5)	Drifting on last step Lacking of counter balance Dropped shoulder Trail leg not counter-balancing	Pulling the ball off target Dropped shoulder Inconsistent release point— lofting or dropping Loses balance	Restore balance line. Develop and maintain counter-balance. Slide straight. Flex sliding knee. Keep trail leg as counter-balance to ball-side.

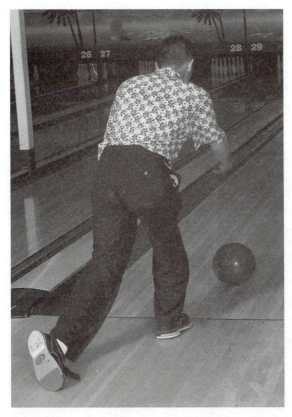

Figure 5.3
Sliding on the wrong foot.

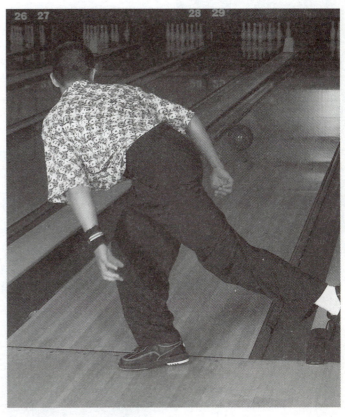

Figure 5.4
Foot turned sideways at the line.

ERROR	CAUSE	EFFECT	CORRECTION
Off-balance forward	Bending too much at waist Over-reaching Steering or guiding ball Lunging	Steering or guiding ball Lunging Lack of lift Late thumb release	Restore balance line. Extending arm only enough to complete pendulum swing. Flex knees. Hold shoulders more upright. Avoid kicking trail leg up in air.
Rearing up	Attempt to achieve lift Attempt to get pin action Insecure thumb grip	Loft of ball Muscled delivery Feel of "losing" ball	Let momentum of ball work. Check size of thumb hole in downswing. Maintain knee bend and balance line at release. Follow-through with arm, not body.
Fouling (Figure 5.6)	Starting position too close Pushaway too long causing steps to be too long Excessive slide Weight back on delivery Excessive approach speed	Loss of pinfall on delivery	Control pushaway. If necessary, move back approximately six inches at a time to reestablish point of origin. Establish balance line. Slow approach tempo.

Figure 5.5
Falling off the balance line.

Figure 5.6
Going over the foul line.

ERROR	CAUSE	EFFECT	CORRECTION
Side-arming	Ball held in middle of body Inside-out or outside-in swing Attempting to "hook" ball	Inconsistent ball path Too much hook Missing target	Position ball in line with right shoulder. Control pushaway. Walk and slide straight to target. Keep elbow close to body during entire swing.
Ball released too soon	Body too straight on release Anxious to put "stuff" on ball Muscling downward Bent too far forward Stiff knee Ball held too loosely Finishing position too high or too low Incorrect ball fit	Lack of lift Ball hooks too much or not enough hook	Maintain natural pendulum swing. Restore balance line. Keep firm grip with all fingers. Restore balance line. Select ball with proper span and hole sizes. Snug thumb hole.
Ball released too late	Overreaching Steering (guiding) ball Thumb hole too tight Too much pitch in thumb hole Attempt to get "lift"	Steering (guiding) ball Skidding Inconsistent ball path Weak ball—no hitting power Loft	Maintain pendulum swing. Make sure thumb hole size and pitch allows free thumb release. Restore balance line. Grip ball firmly but without tension.

Release:

ERROR	CAUSE	EFFECT	CORRECTION
Cut-off armswing (bent elbow) (Figure 5.7 on page 58)	Not extending arm forward Eagerness to apply lift Using forearm too much Improper fit of ball Span too long	Inconsistent ball path and direction Lofting ball	Maintain pendulum swing. Firmness of grip plus pendulum swing will produce desired lift and roll. Maintain straight elbow on follow-through.
Dropped ball	Poor timing Throwing ball into approach or lane Too much weight on ball-side foot Holes too large and/or improper pitches Lack of balance line Incorrect span	Inconsistent ball path and direction	Synchronize movements. Restore balance line. Keep firm grip with all fingers. Hole sizes and pitches should allow ball control to be maintained until released beyond the bottom of pendulum arc. Select ball with the proper span.
Lofted ball	Stiff sliding-side knee Hanging on to ball too long Holes too small and/or too much pitch Attempt to get "lift"	Inconsistent ball path Ball skids too much, little roll or hook	Restore balance line. Maintain pendulum swing. Flex sliding-side knee. Check holes for size and pitch, especially thumb hole. Use less "muscle" at release point.

ERROR	CAUSE	EFFECT	CORRECTION
Not consistent in alignment and height of arm follow-through (Figure 5.8)	Poor timing Lack of balance line Faulty release Over-reaching Exaggerated follow-through (Statue of Liberty) Forced completion of pendulum arc	Forced completion of pendulum arc Ball path and direction inconsistent execution.	Synchronize movements. Restore balance line. Check release. Allow follow-through to be natural continuation of pendulum arc. Follow-through arm directly in front of shoulder.

Overall Delivery:

Too fast	Ball held too high Pushaway too forceful Pushaway too long		Position ball in stance to encourage controlled pushaway and pendulum swing.
	Swing too fast	Poor timing Too much speed on ball	
	Approach too long Bent too far forward	Lack of hook Ball deflects	Decrease size of steps. Develop balance line.
Too slow	Standing too upright Uncertainty Carrying ball Approach too short Pushaway downward	Inconsistent release Too much hook Insufficient speed on ball	Develop pendulum swing. Let swing govern feet. Move point of origin back slightly. Push the ball out in a downward direction and accentuate the pushaway.

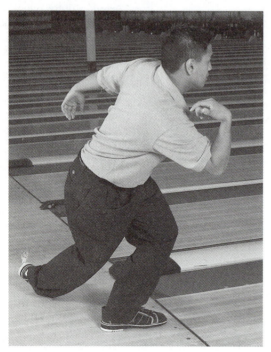

Figure 5.7
Short follow-through, early elbow flex.

Figure 5.8
Sideways follow-through.

ERROR	CAUSE	EFFECT	CORRECTION
Steps too long	Exaggerated pushaway	Approach looks and feels awkward Lack of fluid motion	Shorten steps—synchronize with pendulum swing.
Steps too short	Carrying ball Ball not pushed forward enough Letting footwork govern swing	Letting footwork govern swing Poor timing Approach looks and feels awkward Lack of fluid motion	Develop smooth controlled pushaway. Let pushaway and pendulum swing govern feet.
Ball "double-dribbled" at release	Excessive waist bend	Loss of ball action	Maintain balance line and direction at release. Check knee bend.
Ball rolling over holes	Poor wrist and finger position	Loss of roll and hook	Check fit of ball. Maintain firm wrist and finger position at release. Keep elbow firm during swing.
Drifting	Not aligned properly with target Feeling of too far right or left at point of origin Facing target incorrectly Pushing ball outside or inside shoulder line First step a cross-over or side-step Outside-in or inside-out swing Side-arming in delivery Misdirected follow-through Not keeping eyes on target	Develop outside-in or inside-out armswing Side-arming in delivery Push or pull ball at release Looking at pins to see results	Align ball, shoulder, and target. Push ball straight ahead toward target. Step forward straight ahead. Maintain pendulum swing. Concentrate on target until ball passes over it.

Ball Path and Direction:

ERROR	CAUSE	EFFECT	CORRECTION
Not enough hook	Too much speed Poor timing Overreaching Pushing Steering (guiding) ball Dropping ball Lofting Incorrect hand position Lack of lift Thumb hole too tight Overturn in release Skidding ball Ball too heavy	Lack of hitting power Lack of proper angle of entry into pocket Maximizing deflection	Synchronize movements. Maintain pendulum swing. Keep firm wrist and finger grip. Keep fingers at 4–5 o'clock position throughout swing (generally) Check ball for weight and hook dynamics. Let thumb out of ball first and allow fingers to lift. Decrease approach and ball speed. Use a bowling ball with a duller, more porous surface. Adjust stance and target to the right.
	Poor adjustment to lane conditions	Ball travels through too much oil	Adjust stance and target to the right.

ERROR	CAUSE	EFFECT	CORRECTION
Too much hook	Poor timing Pulling Insufficient ball speed Ball too light Early release Ball rolls too early Outside fingers too far on side of ball Excessive lift and/or excessive turn	Ball rolls too early Lack of accuracy Depending upon the weight of ball—too much angle or too much deflection	Synchronize movements. Maintain pendulum swing. Check firmness of grip and wrist not cupped. Check ball for hook dynamics. Lift through ball not acutely counter-clockwise.
	Poor adjustment to lane conditions	Ball traveling across dry portion of the lane	Adjust stance and target to the left. Use a bowling ball with shinier, less-porous surface.
Inconsistent hook	Hand and wrist positions vary during approaches	Inability to roll ball across target Inconsistent impact points	Maintain firm wrist. Maintain consistent finger position. Deliver ball at same speed every time.
Ball generally too light in pocket	Excessive speed in delivery Ball line too deep Ball line too far outside Overreaching Pushing-steering ball Lack of lift Rearing Skidding ball Inside-out swing Wrap-around swing High backswing Drifting	Lack of striking power Maximum deflection	Control pushaway and maintain pendulum swing. Check starting and finishing position of slide foot to see if delivery foot steps are straight. Check thumb and finger position at release point. Maintain firm grip with wrist and fingers. Check balance line at release. Check position of ball in stance. Increase lift. Adjust starting position and target to the right.
Ball generally too heavy in pocket	Slow ball Ball line too deep Ball line too far outside Pulling ball Rearing Early release Excessive lift Outside-in swing Wrap-around swing Drifting	Excessive split and spare leaves Acute angle of entry	Check starting and finishing position of slide foot to see if delivery foot steps are straight. Control pushaway and maintain pendulum swing. Check thumb and finger position at release point. Maintain firm grip with wrist and fingers. Check balance line at release. Check position of ball in stance. Follow-through in line with shoulder. Avoid rearing up. Check the arm position in stance and direction of pushaway. Adjust starting position and target to the left.

6

3–1–2 Strike Adjustment System

One of the more challenging aspects of the bowling game is adjusting to changing **lane conditions**. Even lanes within the same establishment play differently due to atmospheric conditions, time of day, the quality and amount of play, or the difference in maintenance procedures. Because of these differences in characteristics, the bowling ball may hook more or less from one lane to another. It is the bowler's responsibility to adjust to the lane. As long as the bowler can reasonably deliver the ball consistently in the same way, adjustments can be made.

The **3–1–2 strike adjustment system,** the most fundamental adjustment in bowling, is based on a mathematical computation which will aid in determining how much delivery adjustment is needed. It takes the guesswork out of adjusting the strike ball delivery, but it only applies to the first delivery of a frame.

The adjustment takes place in the delivery stance after judging where the ball is consistently contacting the pins in relation to the head pin. Remember, the second target arrow remains the constant point of aim. The only thing that should be adjusted is the foot position in a new point of origin. The **basic rule of thumb** is to move in the direction of the error or mistake. If you deliver the ball and the ball hooks too much traveling left of the 17th board, move the stance left. If the ball goes too far right, move right.

Figure 6.1
(Right Handers) Pins and corresponding boards.

Figure 6.2
(Left Handers) Pins and corresponding boards.

Before going any further, a quick review is needed.

For Right Handers

- The head pin is on the 20th board.
- The 1–3 pocket is on the 17th board.
- The 3 pin is near the 14th board.
- The Brooklyn pocket is near the 23rd board (Figure 6.1).

For Left Handers

- The head pin is on the 20th board.
- The 1–2 strike pocket is on the 17th board from the left.
- The 3 pin is on the 26th board from the left.
- The crossover pocket of the 1–3 is near the 23rd board from the left (Figure 6.2).

Self Evaluation Questions

1. In a strike ball delivery, if the ball consistently goes left, which direction do you move in the stance? If it goes right?

2. How does the 3–1–2 system work?

3. The following are found on what boards?

    a. 1–3 pocket

    b. 1 pin

    c. 3 pin

    d. Brooklyn pocket

With the previous information in mind, the bowler can make adjustments by determining the number of boards separating the pocket from the actual point of contact of the ball. Specifically, this 3–1–2 system states, **for every 3 boards the ball is off at the pins, move the feet in the stance 2 boards in the direction of the error** (Figures 6.3 and 6.4).

Figure 6.3
The 3–2–1 Strike Adjustment System for right-handers.
(Courtesy of NBC)

For Right Handers

If the ball is properly delivered and rolls over the second arrow but strikes the head pin flush, leaving big splits time after time, the following adjustment should be made. Knowing the head pin is on the 20th board and the 1–3 pocket is on the 17th board, the bowler is able to determine that this ball roll is 3 boards left of the pocket. Using the 3–1–2 formula, move the stance 2 boards to the left (Figure 6.5).

On another day or lane, the ball may be consistently entering the Brooklyn pocket. The Brooklyn pocket is 6 boards to the left of the 1–3 pocket, so the needed adjustment to be made is moving the point of origin 4 boards to the left (Figure 6.6).

And on yet another day or lane, the ball may roll down the lane and contact the 3 pin flush, missing the head pin altogether. The 3 pin is approximately 3 boards away from the pocket, so the adjustment is made by moving the point of origin 2 boards to the right (Figure 6.7).

STRIKE ADJUSTMENT SYSTEM
(Right Handers)

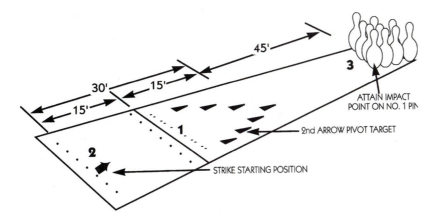

STRIKE ADJUSTMENT SYSTEM
(Left Handers)

Figure 6.4
The 3–1–2 Strike Adjustment System for left-handers.
(Courtesy of NBC)

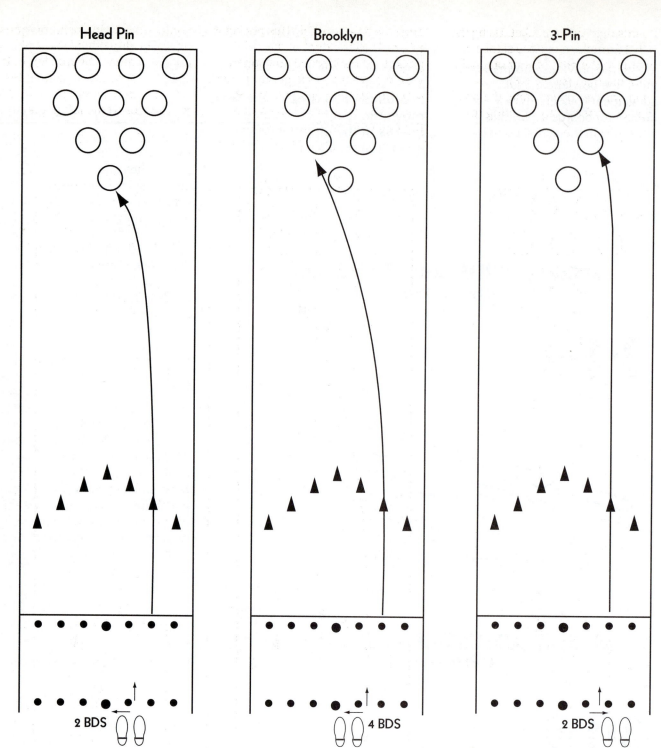

Head Pin

Brooklyn

3-Pin

2 BDS

4 BDS

2 BDS

Figure 6.5
(Right-hand adjustments). If the strike ball consistently hits the head pin flush, move feet in stance *2 boards left in stance*.

Figure 6.6
If the strike ball consistently hits the Brooklyn pocket (1–2 pins), move feet *4 boards to the left in stance*.

Figure 6.7
If the strike ball consistently hits the 3 pin flush, move *2 boards right in stance*. **Remember:** Move in the direction of the error (If ball goes too far left, move left. If ball goes too far to the right, move right).

For Left Handers

If the ball is properly delivered and rolls over the second arrow from the left but strikes the head pin flush, leaving big splits time after time, the following adjustment should be made. Knowing the head pin is on the 20th board and the 1–2 pocket (strike pocket for left handers) is on the 17th board from the left, the bowler is able to determine that this ball roll is three boards right of the pocket. Using the 3–1–2 formula, move the stance 2 boards to the right of your original point of origin (Figure 6.8).

On another day or lane, the ball may be consistently entering the crossover 1–3 pocket. This pocket is 6 boards to the right of the 1–2 pocket, so the needed adjustment would be to move the point of origin 4 boards to the right (Figure 6.9).

And yet, on another day or lane, the ball may roll down the lane and contact the 2 pin flush, missing the head pin altogether. The 2 pin is approximately 3 boards left of the 1–2 pocket so the adjustment is made by moving the point of origin two boards to the left (Figure 6.10).

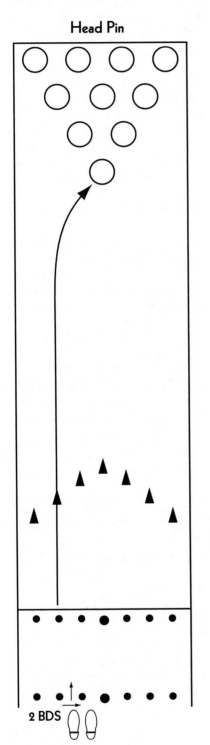

Figure 6.8
(Left-hand adjustments). If the strike ball consistently hits the head pin flush, move *2 boards to the right in stance*.

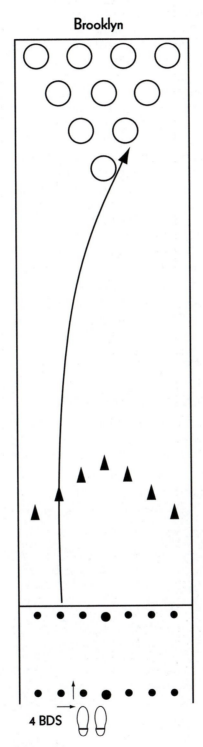

Figure 6.9
If the strike ball consistently crosses over to the Brooklyn pocket (1–3 pins), move *4 boards right in stance*.

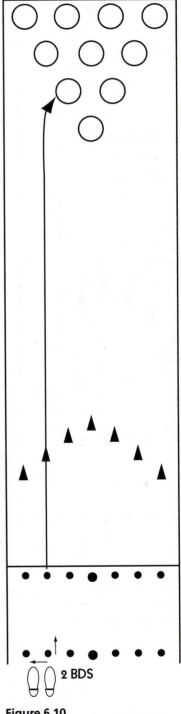

Figure 6.10
If the strike ball consistently hits the 2 pin flush, move *2 boards left in stance*.

This adjustment system will work only when the bowler faces and walks toward the target arrow. This will result in the bowler walking at a slight angle and playing the lane on diagonals. Walking toward the target arrow will put the bowler in the proper delivery position, and will prohibit the bowler from following-through with poor direction or dropping the shoulder in order to hit the target.

Mathematical Formula

How does this system work mathematically? We have already established that it is 75 feet from the third row of locator dots to the head pin. The distance from the starting position to the target arrow (the pivot point) is approximately 30 feet. That leaves a 45 foot spread from the target arrow to the head pin, so the ball has another 15 feet further to roll. Putting this into a ratio, the stance-to-target ratio is 30 feet to 75 feet, with the target pin ratio at 45 feet to 75 feet. Breaking into smaller fractions, it is a ratio of two-fifths to three-fifths, or 2:3. If the bowler makes a two board adjustment in the starting position, and the ball rolls across the same target arrow, the result is a three board change when the ball hits the pins. This is all due to the length of the lane involved and the distance between the starting position, the target, and the pins.

Once the bowler makes an adjustment, it is necessary to turn the body and feet to face the target arrow and to walk toward it during the approach. This will result in a one board change (or adjustment) at the point of release at the foul line. It is 15 feet from the start to the foul line and another 15 feet from the foul line to the target. Thus, if the bowler, for example, adjusts two boards left in the stance, then the sliding foot at release point would actually be one board to the left of the old point of origin.

Words of Advice

When using this system, one must heed a few words of advice. Don't make adjustments on the basis of a single delivery or poor deliveries. Be certain that it was a good delivery and that it did go over the target arrow consistently. Don't confuse "pulling the ball" with too much hook; or following-through toward the right with too little hook.

Additionally, keep in mind that this system works very well if making one or two adjustments (2-to-4 board adjustment in the stance, either left or right). However, if a third adjustment is attempted, the system tends to break down because, at this point, it becomes necessary to also make a target adjustment. Nevertheless, there should be no problem moving a total of 4 boards in either direction.

This system can also be used if the strike ball is hitting light (more on the 3 pin than the 1) or heavy (more on the 1 pin than the 3) by moving half the distance in the stance or one board. Again, this follows the formula since this means the ball is hitting the pocket at the 15.5 board and the 18.5 board, respectively. The error is one-half of the 3 board error, or 1.5 off target. If the bowler uses ratio of 3:2, the feet would be adjusted 1 board in the stance.

Self Evaluation Questions

1. After your foot adjustments in the 3–1–2, in what direction do you take your approach?

2. What stance adjustments must be made if the strike ball consistently hits the following?

   a. Head pin

   b. Heavy on the 3

   c. Heavy on the 1

In a Nutshell:

- The 3–1–2 strike adjustment system is mathematically formulated according to the dimensions of the lane.
- For every 3 boards the ball is off when it hits the pins, move 2 boards in the starting position.
- Move the stance in the direction of the error or mistake. If the ball goes too far to the right, move right or vice versa.
- With this stance, the body and feet must be square to the target, the intended line of ball roll, and *not* the foul line.
- When executed properly, the bowler's slide foot at release point should *not* be on the same board as aligned in the stance. The bowler should have intentionally "drifted" or walked toward the target.
- This system only works within a 4 board stance adjustment in either direction.
- This system works in any proportion of the mathematical ratio.

3–6–9 Spare Conversion System

The 3–6–9 spare system is the most basic of all spare conversion systems. It has been scientifically developed for accuracy and uses a constant target for consistency and ease of learning. It is a system that takes the guesswork out of spare conversions.

Before this spare adjustment system can be implemented, the bowler must be cognizant of the following principles:

The key pin must be identified in all spare conversion attempts.

- If the key pin happens to be one of the strike ball or center of the lane pins, there is no, or very little, adjustment that takes place from the strike ball delivery.
- The basic rule of thumb for pins remaining to the right or left of the center pins is to move the stance origin to the side of the approach area opposite the location of the pins standing (Figures 7.1 and 7.2). If the pins remain standing in the center of

the lane, the strike ball stance and target are used.

The adjustments to pick up pins to the left and right of center are made from two points of origin:

Right Handers:

- All adjustments for pins remaining on the left of center are made from the correct point of origin for the strike ball delivery.
- All adjustments for pins remaining on the right of center are made from the correct point of origin for the 10-pin delivery.

Left Handers:

- All adjustment for pins remaining on the right of center are made from the correct point of origin for the strike ball delivery.
- All adjustments for pins remaining on the left of center are made from the correct point of origin for the 7-pin delivery.

Figure 7.1
A right hander converting a 7 pin.

Figure 7.2
A right hander converting a 10 pin.

Key pin in
2-pin leave

a

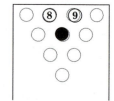

Key pin in
3-pin leave

b

Key pin in baby
4–5 split

c

Key pin in 4-pin
leave with headpin

d

Key pin in splits other
than baby splits

e

Figure 7.3
Key pins for basic spare conversions.

Key Pin Identification

The strike ball point of origin has been established in the previous chapter, so now we need to learn how to locate the key pin. The key pin is the pin that needs to be contacted in order for all other pins to fall. It is the only pin on which to focus attention during a spare conversion. This pin in a 2-pin leave is the closest to the bowler (Figure 7.3A). In a 3-pin cluster, it is the pin in the middle (Figure 7.3B). In a baby split (where the ball can be fitted in between the two pins), it is the pin missing between the 2 pins left standing (Figure 7.3C). If four or more pins are standing and the head pin is one of them, the head pin is the key pin (Figure 7.3D). In a split where the pins are greater than 12 inches apart, the key pin is the pin, either real or imaginary, adjacent to the one closest to you on the outside of the combination (Figure 7.3E).

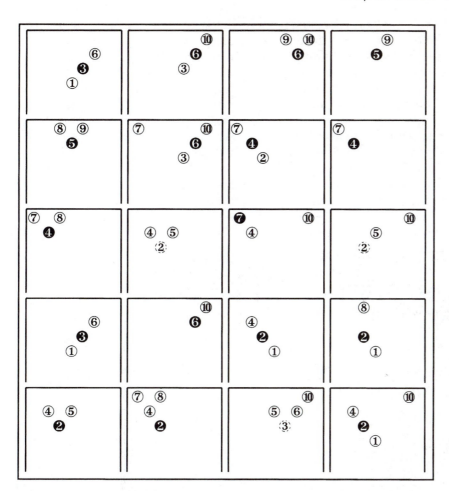

Figure 7.4
Identifying the key pin.

Self Evaluation Question

1. What is the key pin in each of the following?

   a. 2–4–5

   b. 1–3–6

   c. 6–9–10

   d. 9–10

   e. 6–7–10

   f. 2–4–7

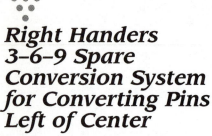

Right Handers 3–6–9 Spare Conversion System for Converting Pins Left of Center

In converting pins to the left of the head pin, the key pin must be located and then, using the rule of thumb, the feet will be moved right of the strike ball origin (Figures 7.5,

and 7.6A, and 7.6B). For each pin to the left of the head pin, the feet will be moved right 3 boards while going over the 2nd arrow from the right. In order to convert the 2-pin, or any combination of the 2-pin (2–4–5, 2–8, 1–2–4, and so on), move the starting stance 3 boards to the right of the strike ball stance, aim for the second target arrow from the right, and walk toward the 2 pin slightly (Figures 7.7A and 7.7B). The 2-pin, or any combination of the 2-pin, will be covered by the ball, providing the delivery is consistent.

To convert the 4-pin, or any 4-pin combination, the bowler must move 6 boards to the right of the strike ball stance, aim for the same second target arrow, and walk toward the 4-pin (Figures 7.8A and 7.8B).

When the 7-pin is left standing, or when it is the key pin, the bowler will move 9 boards to the right of the strike ball stance, aim for the second arrow, and walk toward the 7-pin (Figures 7.9A and 7.9B).

SPARE ADJUSTMENT SYSTEM
(Right Handers)

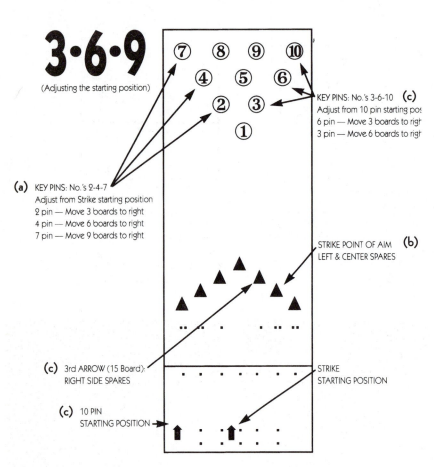

3•6•9
(Adjusting the starting position)

(a) KEY PINS: No.'s 2-4-7
Adjust from Strike starting position
2 pin — Move 3 boards to right
4 pin — Move 6 boards to right
7 pin — Move 9 boards to right

KEY PINS: No.'s 3-6-10 **(c)**
Adjust from 10 pin starting pos
6 pin — Move 3 boards to right
3 pin — Move 6 boards to right

STRIKE POINT OF AIM **(b)**
LEFT & CENTER SPARES

(c) 3rd ARROW (15 Board):
RIGHT SIDE SPARES

STRIKE
STARTING POSITION

(c) 10 PIN
STARTING POSITION

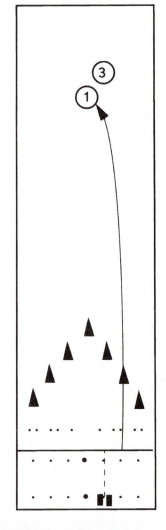

Figure 7.5
(Right handers) Spare Adjustment System.
a. The 3–6–9 adjustment for left-side spares.
b. The spare angle and target arrow used for the 10 pin.
c. The 3–6 adjustment made for right-side spares.

Figure 7.6A and 7.6B
Right-hander's strike point of origin.

Point of origin

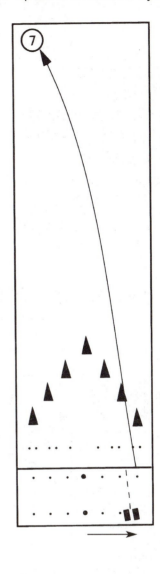

Figure 7.7A
2-Pin spare—Move 3 boards to the right from the strike ball point of origin.

Figure 7.8A
4-Pin spare—Move 6 boards to the right from the strike ball point of origin.

Figure 7.9A
7-pin spare—Adjust 9 boards to the right from the strike ball point of origin.

Figure 7.7B
2-Pin spare—Adjust 3 boards to the right from the strike ball point of origin.

Figure 7.8B
4-pin spare—Adjust 6 boards to the right from the strike ball point of origin.

Figure 7.9B
7-pin spare—Adjust 9 boards to the right from the strike ball point of origin.

Self Evaluation Question

1. What will your point of origin be in order to convert the following key pins?

    a. 4 pin

    b. 7 pin

    c. 2 pin

    d. 8 pin

    e. 5 pin

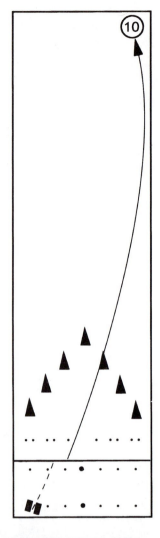

Figure 7.10A
Right-hander's 10-pin point of origin.

Remember: If the bowler walks toward the key pin, it will put the body at a slight angle to the foul line. This is the only way these spare adjustments will work properly. The shoulders are square to the target arrow and the key pin, not to the foul line.

The importance of delivering and rolling the ball the same way, over the same target arrow, changing the point of origin, cannot be overemphasized in the 3–6–9 system. This only changes the approach angle slightly and allows the conversion of spares without changing the armswing or movement toward the foul line.

Right Handers 3–6–9 Spare Conversion System for Converting Pins Right of Center

Conversion of right-side spares uses the same theory as just discussed; however, the point of origin and the target changes. Instead of using the strike ball origin, one now adjusts from the 10-pin point of origin,

always using the 3rd target arrow from the right (Figure 7.5).

To find the point of origin for the 10 pin, the stance, using the left foot as a guide, should be at the place near the left edge of the lane at least 15 boards left of center (Figures 7.10A and 7.10B). Draw an imaginary line through the third arrow from the right to the 10 pin. Still on the left, walk toward the 10 pin and deliver the ball in the same place. If the ball goes into the channel, move a board or two to the right. If the ball goes too far to the left of the 10 pin, move a board or two to the left. When the correct adjustments have been made, and when it is certain the right origin board has been found for the 10 pin, the spare adjustments for the other pins on the right of center may be made. Again using the rule of thumb, for the right of center spares, find the key pin and then move 3 boards to the right of your 10-pin stance for each pin away from the 10 pin that the key pin is located. Go over the 3rd arrow from the right.

To convert the 6 pin, or any combination of the 6 pin, move three boards right of the 10-pin origin point, face the third target arrow, walk and swing toward the 6 pin (Figures 7.11A and 7.11B).

Figure 7.10B
Right-hander's 10-pin point of origin.

For the 3-pin conversion, or any combination of the 3 pin, move 6 boards to the right of the 10-pin point of origin, face the target arrow, walk and swing toward the 3 pin (Figures 7.12A and 7.12B).

A spare conversion involving the 1 pin or the 5 pin is the basic strike ball. No adjustment from your strike ball point of origin or target is necessary.

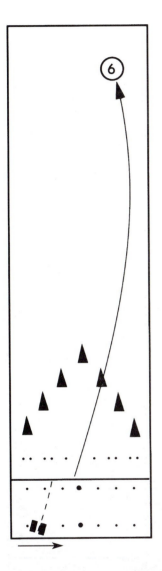

Figure 7.11A
6 pin—Move 3 boards right of 10-pin point of origin.

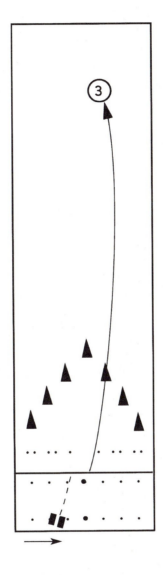

Figure 7.12A
3 Pin—Move 6 boards right of 10-pin point of origin.

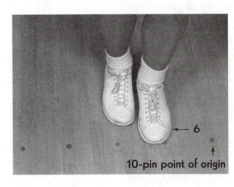

Figure 7.12B
3 pin—Adjust 6 boards to the right from the 10-pin point of origin.

Figure 7.11B
6 pin—Adjust 3 boards to the right from the 10-pin point of origin.

Self Evaluation Question

1. What will be your point of origin in order to convert the following key pins?

    a. 5 pin

    b. 6 pin

    c. 9 pin

    d. 10 pin

    e. 3 pin

Left Handers 3–6–9 Spare Conversion System for Converting Pins Right of Center

On spare conversions where the pins standing are right of the head pin, the key pin must be located and then, using the 3–6–9 rule of thumb, the feet will be moved left of the strike ball origin (Figure 7.13, 7.14A and 7.14B). For each pin to the right of the head pin, the feet will be moved left three boards and go over the second arrow from the left. In order to convert the pin or any combination of the 3 pin (3–5–10, 3–5–6, 1–3–6, 3–9, and so on), move the starting stance 3 boards to the left of your strike ball stance, aiming for the second arrow from the left, and walking slightly toward the 3 pin (Figures 7.15A and 7.15B).

To convert the 6 pin or any 6 pin combination, the bowler must move 6 boards left of the strike ball stance, aiming for the same second arrow from the left, and walking toward the 6 pin (Figures 7.16A and 7.16B).

When the 10 pin is left standing, the bowler will move nine boards left of the strike ball stance, aim for the second arrow from the left, and walk toward the 10 pin (Figures 7.17A and 7.17B).

SPARE ADJUSTMENT SYSTEM
(Left Handers)

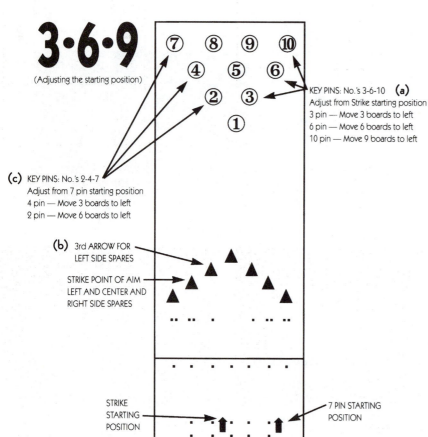

3·6·9
(Adjusting the starting position)

KEY PINS: No.'s 3-6-10 **(a)**
Adjust from Strike starting position
3 pin — Move 3 boards to left
6 pin — Move 6 boards to left
10 pin — Move 9 boards to left

(c) KEY PINS: No.'s 2-4-7
Adjust from 7 pin starting position
4 pin — Move 3 boards to left
2 pin — Move 6 boards to left

(b) 3rd ARROW FOR LEFT SIDE SPARES

STRIKE POINT OF AIM LEFT AND CENTER AND RIGHT SIDE SPARES

STRIKE STARTING POSITION

7 PIN STARTING POSITION

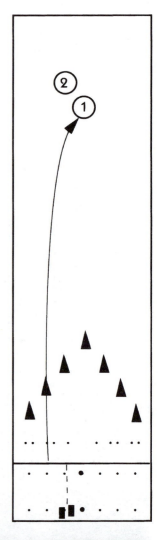

Figure 7.14A
Strike ball.

Figure 7.13
Left-hander's Spare Adjustment System.
a. 3–6–9 adjustment for the right-side spares.
b. The spare angle and target arrow for the 7 pin.
c. The 3–6 adjustment for left-side spares.

Figure 7.14B
Left-hander's strike point of origin.

Point of origin

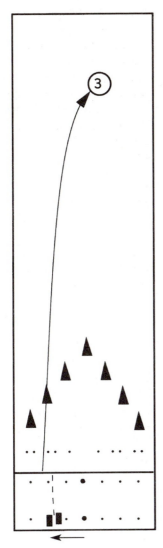

Figure 7.15A
3-pin—Move 3 boards left of the strike ball point of origin.

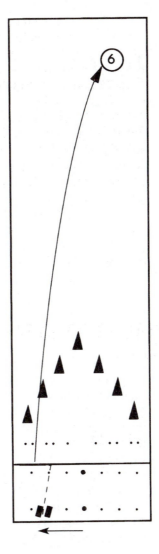

Figure 7.16A
6 Pin—Move 6 boards left of strike ball point of origin.

Figure 7.17A
10 Pin—Move 9 boards left of strike ball point of origin.

Figure 7.15B
3 Pin spare—Adjust 3 boards to the left from the strike ball point of origin.

Figure 7.16B
6 Pin—Adjust 6 boards to the left from the strike ball point of origin.

Figure 7.17B
10 Pin—Adjust 9 boards to the left from the strike ball point of origin.

Self Evaluation Question

1. Where will your point of origin be in order to convert the following key pins?

   a. 3 pin

   b. 10 pin

   c. 5 pin

   d. 9 pin

   e. 6 pin

Left Handers 3–6–9 Spare Conversion System for Converting Pins Left of Center

Conversion of left-side spares uses the same theory as just discussed in the spare conversions right of center. However, the point of origin and the target change. Instead of using the strike ball point of origin, a left-handed bowler now adjusts from the 7-pin point of origin, always using the 3rd arrow from the left as the target (Figure 7.13).

To find the point of origin for the 7 pin, the stance, using the right foot as a guide, should be placed near the right edge of the lane, at least 15 boards right of center (Figures 7.18A and 7.18B). Draw an imaginary line through the 3rd arrow from the left to the 7 pin that your ball would likely follow. Still on the right, walk toward the 7 pin and deliver the ball over the third arrow from the left. If the ball goes into the channel, move a board or two to the left. If the ball goes too far to the right of the 7 pin,

move a board or two to the right. When the correct adjustments have been made, and when it is certain the right origin board has been found for the 7 pin, the spare adjustments for the other pins left of center may be made. ***Rule of thumb:*** For the left-of-center spares, find the key pin and move 3 boards left from the 7-pin stance for each pin away from the 7 pin the key pin is located. Go over the 3rd arrow from the left.

To convert the 4 pin, or any combination of the 4 pin, move 3 boards left of the 7-pin point of origin, face the third target arrow from the left, walk and swing toward the 4 pin (Figures 7.19A and 7.19B).

For the 2-pin conversion, or any combination of the 2 pin, move 6 boards left of the 7-pin point of origin, face the 3rd arrow from the left, walk and swing toward the 2 pin (Figures 7.20A and 7.20B).

A spare conversion involving the 1 or 5 pin is the basic strike ball. No adjustment from your strike ball stance is needed.

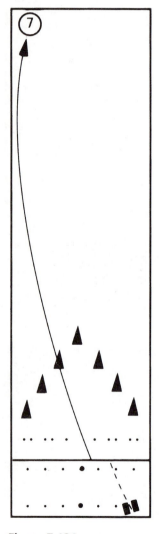

Figure 7.18A
7-pin point of origin and third arrow.

7-pin point of origin

Figure 7.18B
Left-hander's 7-pin point of origin.

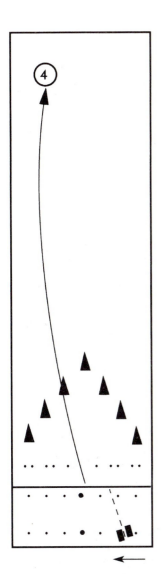

Figure 7.19A
4 Pin—Move 3 boards left of 7-pin point of origin.

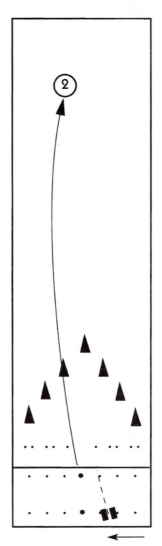

Figure 7.20A
2 Pin—Move 6 boards left of 7-pin stance.

Figure 7.20B
2 Pin—Adjust 6 boards to the left from the 7-pin point of origin.

Figure 7.19B
4 Pin—Adjust 3 boards to the left from the 7-pin point of origin.

Self Evaluation Question

1. Where will your point of origin be in order to convert the following key pins?

   a. 7 pin

   b. 4 pin

   c. 2 pin

   d. 8 pin

In A Nutshell:

By using this 3–6–9 formula, spare conversions become simple and almost automatic. Remember these basic points while using the 3–6–9 adjustment system:

Right Handers:

- Locate the key pin.
- For spare leaves to the left of center, your point of aim is the second target arrow from the right. For spare leaves on the right, focus on the third target arrow from the right.
- For a leave to the left of center, adjust your starting position by moving 3, 6, or 9 boards to the right of your strike ball point of origin. Do this in accordance with your key pin.
- For a leave on the right side of the lane, find the key pin and adjust to this pin by moving either 3 or 6 boards to the right of your 10-pin point of origin.
- Always walk toward the key pin and deliver the ball in the same manner as the strike ball. If delivered properly, the shoulders will be square to the target and

not to the foul line. The footwork should be crossing the approach area at a slight diagonal.

Left Handers:

- Locate the key pin.
- For spare leaves to the right of center, your point of aim is the second target arrow from the left. For spare leaves to the left of center, your target arrow is the third arrow from the left.
- For a leave right of center, adjust your starting position by moving 3, 6, or 9 boards to the left of your strike ball point of origin and go over your second board from the left. Do this in accordance with your key pin.
- For a leave on the left side of the lane, find the key pin and adjust to this pin by moving either 3 or 6 boards left of your 7-pin point of origin and go over the third target arrow from the left.
- Always walk toward your key pin and deliver the ball in the same manner as the strike ball. If delivered properly, the shoulders will be square to the target and not the foul line. The footwork should be crossing the approach area at a slight diagonal.

"If All Else Fails" Addendum

Right Handers' Alternative Method of Converting Spares to the Right of Center

In the case where a bowler cannot grasp the above 3–6–9 method of converting spares that are to the right of center, an alternative method is being presented. Instead of making the adjustments from the 10-pin stance and going over the third arrow as previously stated in this chapter, try moving the stance to the left of your strike ball stance 9–12 or 15 boards while moving your target to the third arrow from the right. This would be your new formula:

To pick up the 3 pin or 9 pin, move 9 boards to the left of your strike ball stance and go over the third arrow from the right (Figure 7.21A).

To pick up the 6 pin, move 12 boards to the left of your strike ball stance and go over the third arrow from the right (Figure 7.21B).

To pick up the 10 pin, move 15 boards to the left of your strike ball stance and go over the third arrow from the right (Figure 7.21C).

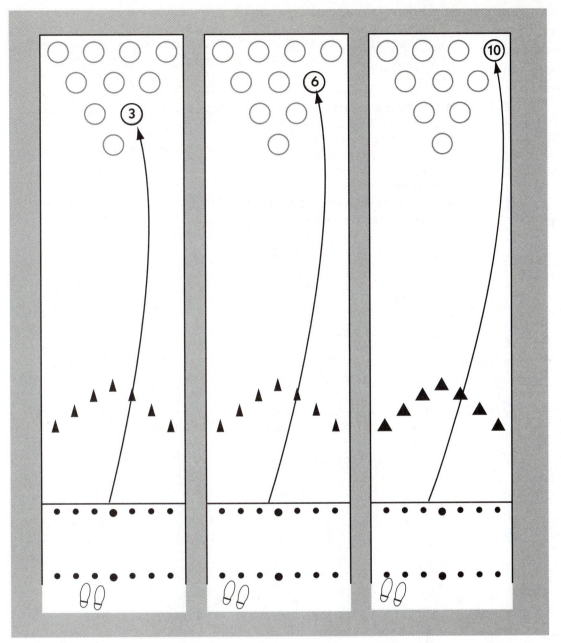

Figure 7.21A
3 Pin—Move 9 boards left of strike ball point of origin—Use third arrow.

Figure 7.21B
6 Pin—Move 12 boards left of strike ball point of origin—Use third arrow.

Figure 7.21C
10 Pin—Move 15 boards (3 dots) to left of strike ball point of origin—Use third arrow.

Left Handers' Alternative Method of Converting Spares to the Left of Center

In the case where a bowler cannot grasp the above 3–6–9 method of converting spares that are to the left of center for left handers, an alternative method is being presented. Instead of making the adjustments from the 7-pin stance as previously stated in the chapter, try moving the stance to the right of your strike ball 9–12 or 15 boards while moving your target to the third arrow from the left. This would be your new formula:

To pick up the 2 or 8 pin, move 9 boards to the right of your strike ball stance and go over the third arrow from the left (Figure 7.22A).

To pick up the 4 pin, move 12 boards to the right of your strike ball stance and go over the third arrow from the right (Figure 7.22B).

To pick up the 7 pin, move 15 boards to the right of your strike ball stance and go over the third arrow from the right (Figure 7.22C).

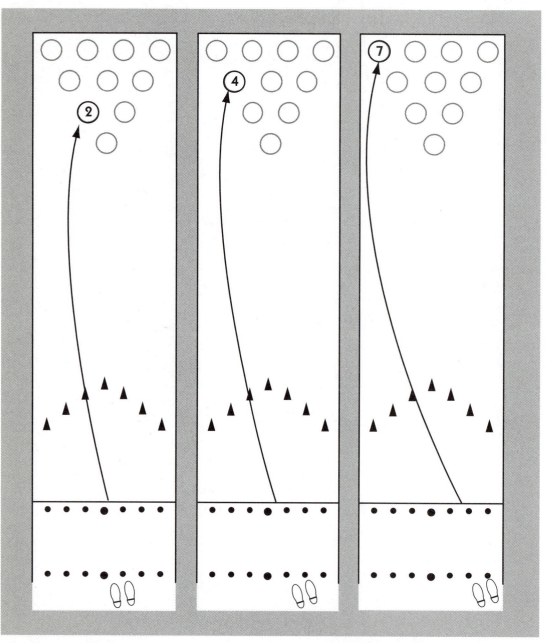

Figure 7.22A
2 Pin—Move 9 boards to right of strike ball point of origin—Go over third arrow.

Figure 7.22B
4 Pin—Move 12 boards to right of strike ball point of origin—Go over third arrow.

Figure 7.22C
7 Pin—Move 15 boards to the right of strike ball point of origin—Go over third arrow.

Bowling for Those with Special Needs

In recent years, enormous strides have taken place in our society to provide recreational services for our special populations. Two special needs groups will be addressed in this chapter of the bowling text—the senior bowler and those with disabilities.

The Senior Bowler

Due to better health care and active lifestyles, the fastest growing group of those with special needs in the United States is the senior citizen. Our seniors are now a very physically active group. Recreational services for this population have grown dramatically in the past decade, providing them with a variety of activities to meet their needs, interests, and abilities (Figure 8.1).

One of the best lifetime activities that has ease of modification, if needed, is the sport of bowling. A variety of bowling activities and programs are readily available for the senior. The following are some tips for the senior bowler.

Tips for the Senior Bowler

Often a senior bowler has a need to work around physical impairments, injuries, phobias, and misconceptions. Sticking to the fundamentals of an activity is not always possible, so adjustments need to be made, taking into account what the bowler physically can or cannot do. Emphasis should be placed on the bowler's strengths (e.g., improving the follow-through when the knee bend cannot be achieved). Also, consideration must be given to the number of games that a senior can bowl at one time (three may be too many). Some special tips for the senior bowler include:

1. Select a bowling ball that is not too heavy. It is better to use a ball that is too light than one that

Figure 8.1
Seniors can find physical activity and enjoyment in bowling.

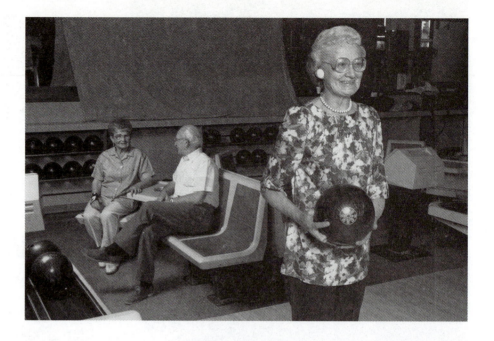

Figure 8.2
Remember to pick the ball up from the return with both hands and face the pins.

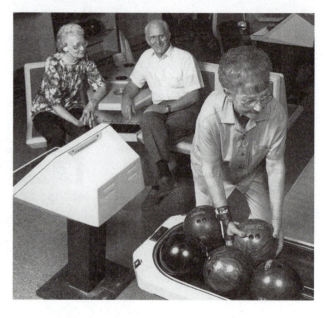

is too heavy in order to keep from tiring too fast. Even if a bowler has bowled for many years, it is important to decrease the weight of the ball to help maintain a consistent ball speed. Often seniors have difficulty acknowledging that they need to decrease ball weight (Figure 8.2).

2. It is strongly advised that seniors use a conventional grip and avoid a fingertip grip. There is less physical strain on the hand using a conventional grip (Figure 8.3).

3. For physical impairments involving the hand, extra holes should be drilled in the ball for gripping purposes. This does not create an illegal bowling ball, as the rules of ABC allow for as many holes to be drilled in the ball as required for gripping purposes. The bowler may sacrifice lift on the ball, but would gain better control of the ball at the release point.

4. For a newcomer to bowling, it would be best to concentrate on a one- or two-step approach.

Often seniors have difficulty in coordinating the armswing with the footwork. By taking fewer steps, effort can be placed on the pendulum swing and release, eliminating thoughts about footwork. A zero-step approach can be employed if there are serious leg or back problems. However, in all of these adjustments, a lack of speed could be a potential shortcoming (Figure 8.4).

Figure 8.3
A senior should use a fingertip grip
only if his or her skill and physical
capabilities allow.

Figure 8.4
Taking fewer steps and starting the
approach closer to the foul line can
help coordination.

5. If the swing and release can
be mastered, then a four-step
approach could be tried.

6. A common problem is an
inability to bend the knees at the
foul line. If this is the case, the
bowler should lean forward more
at the release point to avoid lofting
the ball. Without knee bend, there
is greater tendency to turn the
shoulders and hips away from the
target and to pull the ball across
the body at release. To counteract
this tendency, the bowler needs to
focus on a straight armswing and
follow-through down the lane to
the target (Figure 8.5).

7. A key point for seniors is to
learn how to adjust to lane
conditions. Most tend to roll the
ball very slowly, which allows the
lane to have more time to take
the ball away from its intended
path. To compensate for this lack
of speed, the bowler must be
especially conscious of turning
the body to face the target or the
intended objective.

Figure 8.5
Leaning forward more can help
a senior who has difficulty with
knee bend.

8. Emphasis must be placed on the follow-through. The follow-through must always go in the same direction and to the same level (Figure 8.6).

9. In terms of selecting a target, a senior bowler can still use the dots and arrows that other bowlers use along with the strike and spare adjustment systems. However, it is not an error to be a pin bowler. If this is the case, the bowling shoulder needs to be aligned and turned in the direction of the objective (Figure 8.7).

10. For those with vision problems, using the dots which are seven feet forward of the foul line could be helpful for a closer aiming point. However, the closer one's target, the greater the tendency to bend too much from the waist and have a low follow-through.

11. For a senior who is just beginning to bowl, it is best to deliver the ball so that the thumb points toward the pins (Figure 8.8). The attempt here is to roll a straight ball and to avoid too much roll or hook to the left or to the right. Because of the usual lack of speed, the bowler needs to concentrate on keeping the swing and ball "on line." A hook ball is not a necessity.

Figure 8.6
A consistent follow-through is a key to accuracy.

Figure 8.7
Whichever target is chosen, keep the eyes focused on that target throughout the approach and delivery.

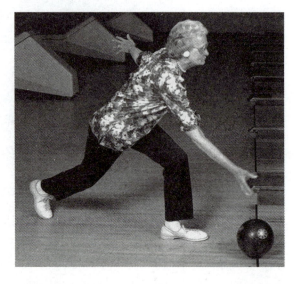

Figure 8.8
Delivering the ball with the thumb pointing toward the pins helps the ball stay on course.

12. To increase consistency, upon the release of the ball, the senior should be conscious of trying to keep the body as still as possible. The only thing that should move is the arm traveling into its natural follow-through. This tip assists in maintaining balance and concentrating on the target.

13. Often with seniors, the conventional "rules" concerning fundamentals do not apply. The "rules" need to be bent to overcome a lack of stamina and There are a variety of disabling conditions, and it would be impossible to cover all of these conditions and the bowling adaptations that would have to be made for treating the uniqueness of each. This would be another book in itself. So it is the authors' intent in this section to give a general overview of guidelines that may benefit those with disabilities and those assisting them.

strength. There is often a need for individual adjustments and "styles" to counteract physical difficulties (Figures 8.9 and 8.10).

Bowling for Those with Disabilities

In recent years, our society has made a concerted effort to bring people with disabilities into the mainstream and into recreational activities. Many of those with disabilities will be able to enjoy the game of bowling without any modifications. Others may need assistance with equipment, or modifications must be made and provided. With the movement of inclusion, many bowling establishments have encouraged those with disabilities to enjoy the challenge of bowling by providing an environment with adaptive devices and equipment to meet the needs of these special bowlers.

Guidelines for Those with Disabilities

1. Select a bowling ball that is not too heavy.

2. A bowling ball with a conventional grip is advised.

3. A one- or two-step approach may be acceptable in many cases.

4. A straight ball release is encouraged for many, but a hook ball is still desirable in many instances.

5. Emphasis is on the delivery and follow-through. Emphasize leaning forward and placing the ball on the lane and following through completely toward the target.

6. Pin bowling may take the place of spot or target bowling. However, if possible, incorporate spot bowling into the bowling fundamentals.

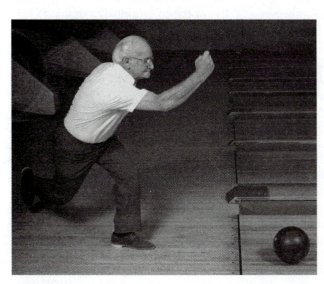

Figure 8.9
This style allows for a short slide.

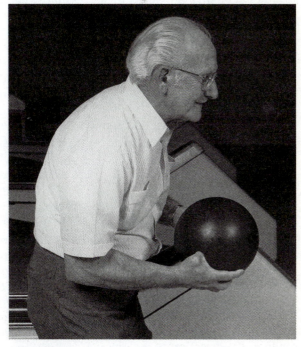

Figure 8.10
This senior finds less strain on his arms by holding the ball centered in the stance.

7. In order to have a measure of success, adaptive devices and equipment are occasionally available at the bowling establishment.

8. Make sure that only one player at a time is on the approach. When not bowling, stay in the settee area.

9. Keep the hands away from the ball return, especially where the ball pops up.

Guidelines for Instructing Those with Disabilities

1. It would be highly advisable to have one-to-one assistance while keeping the groups small.

2. Determine the abilities of each individual and identify the needs and realistic goals for each.

3. In reaching these goals, develop a simple plan of attack and then keep things simple.

4. Keeping things fun is important as ample practice is given to each segment of the skill.

5. Modifications of the game may occur, but most want to play the game/activity the way everyone else does.

6. Each will have a level where he or she is functioning. Many will have to start at the lowest skill level, whereas many may be at a higher level.

7. Each needs to have maximum activity with a minimum of passive time.

8. Each needs praise and lots of celebration!

Examples of adaptive bowling equipment include handle-grip bowling balls where the handles automatically retract into the ball upon delivery; bowling rails to guide the visually impaired; adjustable ball release bowling ramps where the ball is placed atop and then pushed down in the direction of the pins;

and channel bumpers to prevent balls from entering the channel while traveling toward the pins.

For those who do not need adaptive equipment and would like to enjoy the game of bowling on their own but may need slight modifications, we suggest following the previous guidelines written for the senior bowler. By choosing the suggestions that pertain directly to your needs, you will be able to enjoy an afternoon of bowling at your favorite establishment. (For additional information for teaching bowling to the disabled, see the Instructor's Manual.)

Bowling and Pregnancy

There is no reason why a pregnancy should interrupt the enjoyment of the game of bowling. However, it is strongly advised that pregnant bowlers get a physician's release before engaging in the sport of bowling. Most bowlers will very likely be granted this permission and will be able to continue bowling throughout the pregnancy unless there are complications associated with the pregnancy. It is possible during the last month or two that fatigue and the tired back syndrome may limit the bowling of some.

As a pregnant woman engaging in the activity of bowling, there will be a few physical changes that may affect bowling. First of all, the vertical balance line may be slightly skewed, finding the bowler more upright or leaning slightly backward in the approach and delivery. To counter this, it is important to accentuate the arm going farther out toward the target arrow so the release of the ball is farther out on the lane than what seems natural.

Secondly, the legs will have a tendency to tire more easily. Those taking the game seriously may need

to do additional leg strengthening exercises. If the legs do get tired during the games, the knee bend at the release point will be less. Therefore, it is really necessary that the arm again reach out as far as possible to the target to help counter the more upright position of the bowler at the time of the delivery.

Probably the most important element that can be stressed for a pregnant bowler is to guard against additional back pain while participating in bowling. Several suggestions are in order to assist in this endeavor: (1) Avoid carrying bowling equipment long distances. It is advised that a bowler get a bag that has wheels. (2) Always pick up a bowling ball, whether from the bag, racks, or ball return, with hands around the ball and knees bent. Use the straightening of the knees to lift the ball and not the back. (3) When delivering the ball, bend those knees! This will get the body lower on the delivery and will assist in taking the strain of the weight of the ball away from the back.

There is also a possibility that the swing may be affected due to the pregnancy. It is advised that, in the stance, the ball be held slightly off to the side (rather than at the center of the body) to emphasize that the pushaway be in line with the ensuing pendular swing. This should keep everything in a straight line going toward the target arrow.

There is no reason that a pregnant woman cannot enjoy the sport of bowling. Many women will find that they actually will improve their averages during this time, possibly due to a slower more cautious foot speed on the approach, and greater concentration on the balance at the line. Others will find it a bit more challenging. Regardless, the excitement and social aspects of bowling will remain. So after your physician's clearance, go for it!

9

The Modern Bowling Environment and Twenty-first Century Technology

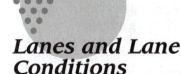

The entire world has been affected by the rapid changes in technology and the development of new materials. Bowling is no exception. In the last twenty years, many changes have taken place in the game of bowling. These changes range from synthetic pins and lanes to new ball surfaces that are capable of being adjusted to the particular lane conditions and oiling systems. The traditional wooden lanes and familiar balls are rapidly disappearing. With the modern changes, bowlers must be prepared (both physically and mentally) to face a bowling environment that may have greater variations and pose new challenges. In this chapter, we hope to give you a glimpse of the modern bowling environment and many of the changes that may be occurring as we enter the twenty-first century.

Lanes and Lane Conditions

Whether the lanes are wooden or synthetic, one of the most crucial variables a bowler must deal with is the variation in lane conditions from lane to lane, day to day, and from establishment to establishment. Lane conditions will even change from the start of a bowling session to the end. The capability of a bowler to make adjustments to correspond with the lane condition at the time will determine the difference between a good performance and a bad performance. Since we have previously indicated several adjustment systems that can be used to adjust to the varying lane conditions, a little information on lane conditions may prove helpful at this time.

As you may guess, the bowling lane surface is subject to a considerable amount of daily play and "wear and tear" on the lane. To minimize the "wear and tear," to equalize lane conditions, and to prevent damage to the surface of the lanes, bowling establishments carefully maintain the lane surfaces. Most establishments care for their lanes on a daily basis. A very thin coat of oil-based "dressing" is applied to the lane surface that helps protect the lane from the balls traveling on it, somewhat as a motor oil protects a car's engine. Oiling machines are now very high tech. They operate on the same principle as an ink-jet printer in that the volume and pattern of oil placed on each single board is predetermined through a computer-type program. In modern bowling establishments, there are two commonly used oiling patterns, commonly known as the Christmas Tree Pattern and the Top Hat Pattern. Each of these patterns will have a different effect on a bowling ball traveling toward the pins. It is advised that bowlers check with their usual bowling establishment, which can provide more in-depth knowledge as to which pattern they are using and how it is applied. This knowledge can then be used in adjusting ones point of origin or point of aim.

Fast Lanes

With the different application systems, amounts of oil, and patterns of lane oiling, we find lanes that will vary a great deal which will affect the ball roll. The greater the quantity of oil applied to the lane, the more the ball tends to skid on its path to the pins. Because of the skid of the ball, it will not "grab" or hook soon enough for the proper angle of entry into the pins. This is usually called a **"fast lane"** or **"oily lane."** Adjustments must take place to enable the ball to break sooner, which is usually done by moving the point of origin in your stance farther right (right handers) or farther left (left handers) (see Chapter 6—3-1-2 Strike Adjustment).

Slow or Hooking Lanes

The lane with less oil, called a **"slow"** or **hooking lane,** allows the ball to hook more. It actually skids less, which allows the ball to begin its roll sooner on the lane. The angle of entry into the pocket generally needs to be decreased by the bowler on this type of lane, so the adjustment for a right-handed bowler would be to generally move his or her point of origin slightly to the left, whereas a left-handed bowler would move his or her point of origin slightly to the right (see Chapter 6—3-1-2 Strike Adjustments).

Today's Lanes

According to the American Bowling Congress, today's lanes must have a minimum of three "units" of dressing applied across the lane for any distance that the lane is dressed. The general effect of this rule should be that the bowler may feel that the lane is oilier and that the ball does not hook as much. It is the bowler's ability to adapt to changing lane conditions that will determine the eventual game score. This process is called "reading the lane" to determine just what adjustments in the target or point of origin may be necessary. It must be remembered that the approach, armswing, and delivery should remain consistent no matter what the lane conditions are like. The correct adjustment to the appropriate strike line will mean the difference between a successful performance or a frustrating one.

Newest Trends in Lanes Found in Twenty-first Century Bowling Establishments

- Even though about 60 percent of the bowling lanes are still made of wood, all recently installed lanes are synthetic and have a laminate surface.

- The new synthetic Brunswick lanes have an additional marking on the lane to assist the "modern" player. Two dark boards (each about 3 feet long) have been added about two-thirds of the way down the lane (or about 40 feet). One is placed on the right and the other on the left. The purpose of these additional targets is to assist the modern player in judging the **"break point"** (the point where the ball stops sliding and starts its move to the pins—usually the widest point in the ball path) (Figure 9.1). These extra boards are used for targeting—to determine when and where the ball hooks.

- **"Bumpers,"** which are fillers in the channels (gutters) used by very young bowlers and those with special needs, are now built into the lanes. The bumpers rotate up into the gutters, preventing gutter balls and allowing everyone to enjoy knocking down pins.

- "Astro Bowling," where lanes actually glow due to an ultraviolet additive to the lane dressing, is popular now in recreational bowling.

- ABC/WIBC has developed a new program called "Sport Bowling" where lane conditions and equipment are more controlled with the purpose of placing more emphasis on a bowler's advanced skill. This is an attempt to decrease the assistance given bowlers from the lane condition and high tech bowling balls. In the United States, leagues are being formed which will bowl on "Sport Bowling" lane conditions. Both the PBA and PWBA (professional bowler's associations) hold their tournaments on these lane conditions, along with all major international amateur organizations and championships.

Figure 9.1
Breaking point in a ball roll.

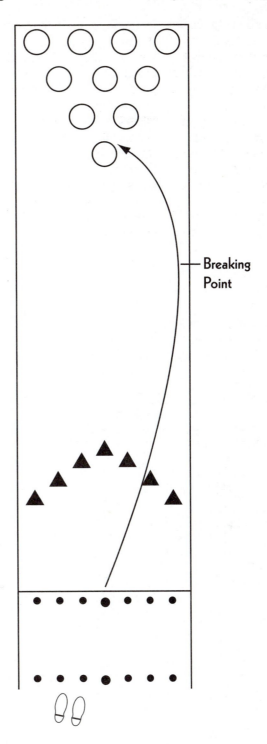

Breaking
Point

- Under "Sport Bowling" conditions, shot-making is at a premium and a bowler is unable to get away with inconsistencies. Absolute command of one's game is needed. This move is meant to try to bring credibility and shot-making (different from accuracy) back to bowling.
- On a "Sport Bowling" lane, the lane conditions can vary a great deal due to the quantity and length of dressing down the lane. However, there may be no more than a 2:1 ratio of dressing anywhere on the lane side-to-side.
- A recreational bowler playing on sport bowling conditions can expect a 20–25 pin drop in his or her average. If a "sport bowler" has established an average on sport bowling lanes, the ABC/WIBC has created a chart

(Figure 9.2) for this bowler to use to determine his or her equivalent adjusted average for recreational bowling. For example, if one who bowls in a "Sport Bowling" league has an average of 170, this average will be adjusted to 188 in a recreational league. A bowler cannot have an average adjusted downward (from recreational to sport); only upward (from sport to recreational).

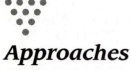

Approaches

Today's synthetic lanes may find bowlers sensing that the approaches feel different. The approaches may feel more slippery than normal, or depending upon climate and humidity, they may feel stickier. Many of today's bowlers are electing to purchase an elite shoe that has removable/changeable soles and heels which can be used as a method of adjusting to approach conditions. However, the average bowler should be prepared to make his or her own adjustments with his or her shoes in order to compensate. The needed supplies to do this are listed at the end of this chapter.

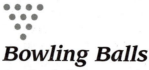

Bowling Balls

Bowling balls have probably gone through the greatest changes in the last twenty years. Everyone is seeking that perfect ball to roll for that changing lane condition. This has resulted in new ball designs and ball covers every couple of years or months. The old rubber and plastic balls have been replaced by urethane and reactive resin balls. The urethane ball is more porous, grabs the lane more, and creates greater hook and hitting power. The reactive resin ball has a "sticky" feel to it and tends to have a greater reaction to the oilier and the dryer parts of the lane. The newest ball on the market at the time of this printing is the resin with additive ball. This ball came on the market in 1998. It has a resin surface with very hard particles of material added to it. These balls tend to have a very

SPORT LEAGUE AVERAGE	ADJUSTED AVERAGE	SPORT LEAGUE AVERAGE	ADJUSTED AVERAGE	SPORT LEAGUE AVERAGE	ADJUSTED AVERAGE
0–129	Same				
130	137	160	175	190	207
131	138	161	176	191	208
132	140	162	176	192	209
133	141	163	177	193	210
134	142	164	179	194	211
135	144	165	180	195	212
136	145	166	182	196	212
137	146	167	184	197	213
138	148	168	186	198	214
139	150	169	187	199	215
140	154	170	188	200	216
141	158	171	189	201	217
142	159	172	190	202	218
143	160	173	192	203	218
144	161	174	194	204	219
145	162	175	195	205	220
146	163	176	196	206	220
147	164	177	197	207	221
148	165	178	198	208	222
149	166	179	199	209	224
150	166	180	200	210	225
151	167	181	201	211	225
152	168	182	201	212	226
153	169	183	202	213	227
154	169	184	203	214	229
155	170	185	204	215	230
156	171	186	205	216	230
157	173	187	205	217	231
158	174	188	206	218	232
159	175	189	207	219 and up	SL Ave+15

Figure 9.2
Sport league average adjustment to standard average chart.

smooth reaction (action is similar to all-season radial tires) and can be polished or sanded for the desired amount of hook (Figure 9.3).

The following is a summary of the four major types of bowling balls currently sought by bowlers:

1. Polyester (plastic)—This ball came on the market in the early 1960s. It is an attractive ball that today comes in many "collector novelty editions" such as Mickey Mouse, sport ball look-alikes (soccer, basketball, baseball), and clear balls with design inserts (flowers, logos, and so on). They range in price from $40 to $140.

2. Urethane—This type of ball came on the market in 1981. It is popular because the desired hook can be altered by simply sanding or polishing the surface. It ranges in price from $80 to $150.

3. Resin—This type of ball came on the market in 1991. The surface of the ball has a "sticky" feel and tends to have a greater reaction to the oilier and the drier parts of the lane. The surface of this ball can also be sanded or polished to the desired ball roll. They range in price from $80 to $280.

4. Resin with Additive—This ball came on the market in 1998. It has the resin surface with very hard particles of material added to it. These balls have a very smooth reaction and can also be polished or sanded for the desired hook. They range in price from $120 to $280.

Note: Bowling establishments may still use the old rubber balls as "house" balls.

The newer balls have resulted in bowlers readily increasing their averages by about 10 pins. The reason for this phenomenon is twofold: the reactive resin cover, as well as the density and shapes of the core of the ball. There are more manufacturers of bowling equipment today than ever before, and each is trying to improve and perfect ball cores. The cores come in ever-increasingly odd shapes and configurations: light bulb-like shapes, mushroom shapes and diamond shapes to name a few (Figure 9.4). They may be symmetrical or asymmetrical. These

Figure 9.3
Bowling balls are made of various materials; their surface can be dull or shiny.

Light Bulb-Type Core

Mushroom-Type Core

Barbell-Type Core

Figure 9.4
Ball cores come in different shapes.

cores, depending upon the design, affect the way the ball will react on the lane and against the pins.

Ball Drilling

The professional who drills the ball must have specialized knowledge in the dynamics of each particular bowler's needs and the bowling ball itself. Professional expertise on the part of the ball driller is an absolute necessity. A bowling ball is no longer a simple round mass impacting ten bowling pins. It has become a dynamic force that overpowers the pins. A ball's deflection has been greatly decreased. The older method of drilling in terms of the old idea of "weights" is no longer influential. In the ball weight method, the ball could only be drilled to create a maximum of a 4–6 inch difference in

hook/roll pattern. However, the owner of a modern day resin with additive ball can change the surface of the ball by sanding or polishing it to the point that the ball can change the hook/roll pattern by feet, not just inches. Therefore, this sanding or polishing of the reactive resin ball with different core structures has taken the place of "weights" or bowling ball "imbalances."

Automatic Scorers

Not every bowling center has automatic scoring devices, but you can readily recognize that a center has the automatic device when there are no lighted overhead projectors. Instead, you will see a television-type screen where the

score is projected over the approach area (Figure 9.5).

Even with a machine that keeps score for the bowler, it is important to learn how to keep score as that knowledge may be crucial in the outcome of a game (e.g., knowing what score a bowler needs in order to win). The major manufacturers have different types of automatic scoring systems (Figure 9.6). Upon entering the bowling center, the personnel at the control desk can provide you with the simple instructions required to make the scorer start. Most automatic scorers can be easily used by following the instructions printed or shown on the screen or the console. Corrections, adding of handicaps, or changes of information can be made manually by the bowler. Assistance can

Figure 9.5
The automatic scoring unit is located in the bowler's settee area.

Figure 9.6
The bowler enters all necessary information into the machine and can also make scoring corrections.

always be obtained from the personnel at the control desk.

Suggested Miscellaneous Bowling Supplies

To be prepared for the great variety of conditions and situations confronting the modern player, a bowler should have some supplies and aids available to him or her. The following supplies should be kept in a player's bowling bag and be available at a moment's notice (Figure 9.7).

For the bowling shoes:

Soapstone—can be applied to the bottom of the bowling shoe and help a bowler to have a smooth slide. Pencil lead or cigarette ashes can eliminate sticking in the same fashion.

Wire brush or coarse sandpaper—to be used to rough up the soles for traction. **Note:** Never use any powder on the bottoms of shoes or on the approaches.

For the hand:

Cotton—for use with skin-patch.
Skin-patch—a liquid to cover blisters, cuts, or tender spots on fingers.
Hand conditioner—to help the hand stay dry and get the same feel of the ball.

This can come in a bag or jar, and be a liquid or a powder.

Towel—to wipe the hand and/or the ball.
Wrist band—to support a weak wrist or lend extra support.
Lip balm or baby powder—for use on the thumb in extreme cases of swelling and a very fast thumb release.

For the ball:

Plastic tape—3/4 or 1" for use in adjusting the size of the thumb or finger holes as necessary. The tape can be cut to any length necessary

and placed along the backside of the holes to make them more snug. The tape can be readily peeled away to make the hole larger.
Scissors—to cut the tape to needed lengths.
Pieces of sandpaper or screen in various grits—to smooth the insides or edges of holes.
Emory board—to file down excessive build-up of calluses.
Fast drying glue—for use on inserts or grips used in thumb or finger holes.
Round file or bevel knife—to repair edges of holes or enlarge them on the spot.
Alcohol—to clean thumb and finger holes from any kind of built-up residue and to clean the outside of the ball from a build-up of dirt or oil. The outside of the ball can only be cleaned prior to or after competition (not during).
Reactive resin ball cleaner—special liquid cleaner for reactive balls which tend to pick up dirt and oil due to their surface "tackiness" (available in pro shops).

Figure 9.7
Some examples of a bowler's necessities.

Having these supplies readily on hand can help a bowler overcome distressful situations and to continue bowling without a severe loss of pinfall. Without them, bowlers could find themselves in a situation where they might as well "call it a day."

The modern bowling environment in the twenty-first century does indeed require more than a ball, shoes, and a bowling lane.

Knowledge and versatility are needed along with the ability to adapt to the ever-changing environments in which we find ourselves.

Appendices

Appendix A

Scoring

The game or line of bowling consists of 10 frames. A bowler gets a maximum of two ball deliveries in each frame to knock all of the pins down. A perfect 300 game is scored by knocking all of the pins down with the first ball roll of each frame.

A typical scoresheet used in bowling is divided into the 10 frames. An accumulation score of each frame is kept in order to come up with the final game score. In the top right corner of each frame is a pair of small boxes, one for each ball roll.

The pinfall on each ball delivery is entered in the little boxes. If a bowler knocks down 7 pins on the first delivery, a 7 is placed in the first box.

If on the second ball, the bowler knocks 2 of the remaining 3 pins down, the 2 is placed in the second little box and the total fall for both balls is recorded in the frame.

If the bowler knocks down all of the pins in a frame in *two* deliveries, a spare is the result and is recorded by placing a diagonal slash (/) in the second little box.

In order to score a spare, the bowler will receive the 10 pins knocked down in that frame plus the pinfall of the next single ball delivery.

10 +   6+3=19

☒ | 63

19

If a bowler knocks down all the pins with the first ball, it is called a strike and is recorded in the first little box as an X. In case of a strike, the second ball is not needed since all of the pins are already knocked down. A bowler who is credited with a strike gets to score the 10 pins he or she knocked down with that ball plus a bonus of the pinfall on the next two deliveries. Therefore, if a strike is recorded, nothing is placed in that frame until that bowler's turn comes up again and he or she rolls the next two balls for the next frame or frames.

10   +10 + 8=28

☒ | ☒ | 8

28

If the bowler records two strikes in a row, it is called a "double." In order to figure the pin count, follow the rule of 10 plus the next 2 balls. In this case, count the 10 pins knocked down by the strike ball, the ten on the first bonus ball, and the eight on the second bonus ball.

10 + 10 + 10=30

☒ | ☒ | ☒

30

If a bowler rolls 3 strikes in a row, it is called a triple or a "turkey." Again, follow the rule of the 10 plus the pin count from the next two ball rolls, which will result in a total of 30.

10 + 10 + 9=29

☒ | ☒ | ☒ | 9 -

30 | 59

Then, using the same formula, figure the score for a double and add to the previous frame score.

10 +   9+0=19

☒ | ☒ | ☒ | 9 -

30 | 59 | 78

Now figure the score for the single strike left.

☒ | ☒ | ☒ | 9 -

30 | 59 | 78 | 87

And finally, add the 9 pin count for the next frame.

If a bowler fails to knock any pins down on a ball roll, a miss (-) is recorded in the respective corner square.

When the pins left following the first delivery constitute a split, a circle is drawn around the number of pins knocked down on that delivery. The pins knocked down on the second ball roll are still recorded in the little right hand box.

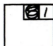

If a bowler fouls on the first delivery of a frame, an F is recorded in the first little box and no pinfall is counted. All of the pins are reset for the second ball delivery. Only the pins knocked down with the second ball are counted; in this case, 6 pins were knocked down.

If, after knocking down pins on the first ball of a frame, a foul is made, an F is recorded in the second little box and only the pinfall of the first ball delivery is counted in that frame.

The 10th frame is the final frame of the game. It is scored exactly as the previously scored frames unless a strike or spare occurs. When a spare occurs in the 10th frame, one bonus ball must be rolled in order to find out how much the spare scores. In this case, 10 (the pins knocked down in the spare) plus the 8 pins knocked down with the bonus ball. The 18-pin count is then added to the total in the 9th frame and placed in the 10th. **That is the end of the game.**

When a strike is recorded in the 10th frame, the bowler must roll two more balls in order to find out how much that strike scores. The score for the last strike (18) is added to the 9th frame score. The total score placed in the 10th frame is the score of the game, and the pinfall from the extra two ball rolls is not added on.

	10	TOTAL
	124	124
	136	260
	103	363

The total column at the end of each line is used to total accumulated game scores. This score constitutes the bowler's series score.

Here is an example of an individual game:

1	2	3	4	5	6	7	8	9	10
7 2	5 ╱	8 ╱	☒	4 3	☒	☒	6 ╱	8 -	☒ ☒ 5
9	27	47	64	71	97	117	135	143	168

How to Calculate an Average

If the total series is divided by the number of games bowled, the bowler's average for the series is obtained (i.e., 363 ÷ 3 = 121). During a competitive season, a bowler keeps a running account of his or her current average. This is accomplished by keeping track of each game bowled and adding it to the cumulative total of games previously bowled. By continually totaling and dividing the total by the number of games bowled, the bowler will find his or her current average. Any extra pins left over (fractions) are dropped from the average.

```
124
136
103
100
152
134
169
122
180
―――
1220 ÷ 9 = 135 average
```

Appendix B

League Bowling

Handicapping

There are basically two major kinds of leagues in bowling: the scratch league and the handicap league. The scratch league merely means the actual scores rolled by the bowler are the scores used in competition. There is no means of equalizing the scores of the bowlers by giving pins to the less-skilled bowler.

The handicap league "gives" pins to less-skilled bowlers in order to equalize their abilities, thus providing better, closer competition. Each league establishes its own handicap formula to be used throughout the season.

There are two main kinds of handicapping: the individual base handicap and the team base handicap. Each league will decide which of these styles of handicapping will be used as well as what base and percentage to use.

The Base Score

The base from which a handicap is figured is usually established by looking at the league's top bowler(s). The base should usually be a little above the top bowler(s) in the league. For leagues with bowlers who average in the 180s and 190s, a 200 base is commonly established. This basically means that a 200 average bowler would be bowling scratch, no handicap. Any bowler under a 200 would get a percentage of the pin difference between his or her average and the handicap base. In a lesser skilled league where the top bowler(s) does not exceed the average of 170 or so, a 180 base may be selected.

The Selected Percentage

To merely subtract a bowler's average from the base score would not be quite fair. Therefore, a designated percentage of the difference between the bowler's average and the base score is identified. The most common percentages are probably 75 and 80 percent, but they may range from 60 to 100.

Figuring Individual Based Handicaps

Some leagues will require that the handicap be figured for each individual on the team. Suppose the league has selected a base score of 180 and an 80 percent handicap figure. The following procedure would be followed to find Sam's handicap per game when he has an average of 140.

Subtract Sam's average from the base score.

Then take 80 percent of that score.

For each game Sam rolls, 32 pins will be added to his score.

$$
\begin{array}{r}
180 \\
-140 \\
\hline
40 \\
\times .80 \\
\hline
32.00
\end{array}
$$

In order to find a team's handicap for each game using this system, each team member's handicap is figured, as was Sam's, and added together.

This team would have a team handicap of 108 pins per game.

Team Base Handicapping

Sometimes it is more convenient to figure the total team handicap all in a single calculation rather than five separate calculations for each of the team members. This is accomplished by finding the team base by multiplying the 180 base score by the number of team members (180 × 5 = 900). This team base score, once found, will remain 900 throughout the season.

Now add all of the team members' averages together, subtract that total from the team base of 900, and take 80 percent of the difference.

Each week the handicap will differ from the week before because the individual averages will change.

		Individual Handicap
Example:	Sam	32
	Jane	40
	Tony	14
	Sue	10
	Jerry	12
		108 pins

		Average	
Example:	Sam	140	900 Team Base
	Jane	130	-765 Team Total Average
	Tony	162	135
	Sue	168	X .80
	Jerry	165	108.00 Pins
		765	

Figuring Marks

In competitive bowling, a player or a team is interested in knowing the status of its score in relation to its opponents' as the game progresses. Instead of totaling each frame, an easy system has been worked out where marks are counted. A strike or a spare is usually referred to as a mark, and each mark is worth a value of 10 pins. By counting the marks in each frame and keeping a running total, the bowler can tell approximately how many pins ahead or behind he or she is in that game. Example:

	1	2	3	4	5	6	7	8	9	10	
TEAM	9 −	5 /	6 2	⑦ 2	F 8	9 /	X	8 1	6 2 X 3 6		
	9	25	33	42	50	70	89	98	106	125	125
A	X	8 1	6 −	X	X	8 −	8 1	5 2	X	7 / 8	
	19	28	34	62	80	88	97	104	124	142	267
(MARKS)	1	2	−	3+1	5	6	7	−	8	10	
TEAM	6 2	9 −	6 /	8 −	X	4 5	8 /	5 3	F 6 9 −		
	8	17	35	43	62	71	86	94	100	109	109
B	6 3	2 /	⑧ −	X	3 3	9 −	4 /	8 −	X	5 / 6	
	9	27	35	51	57	66	84	92	112	128	237
(MARKS)	1	2	3	4	−	6	−	7	8		

By examining the marks in frame 2, Team A has 1 mark more than Team B, which is approximately 10 pins. In the 7th frame, Team A has 7 to Team B's 6 marks, a difference of 1 mark or approximately 10 pins. At that point Team A knows they have about 10 pins more than Team B without looking at the scores. At the end of the game Team A has 2 marks more than Team B, so they will win by approximately 20 pins.

This system is more commonly used in league bowling since team progress is difficult to figure because of the five different scores. After each complete frame, the scorer adds the total marks to that point of the total team.

Mark Guidelines

- To receive a mark, it is necessary for a player to get a strike or a spare.
- To gain 2 marks in a frame, it is necessary for a player to get two strikes in a row.

- Four ways of losing marks are:

1. Following a spare, with the next ball the bowler knocks down fewer than 5 pins.

2. Following a strike, the bowler knocks down less than 5 pins on his or her two attempts.

3. Following a double, the bowler rolls the next ball and knocks down less than 5 pins.

4. Following a double, the bowler knocks down fewer than 5 pins total on two ball deliveries. *Loss of 2 marks.*

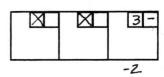

Figuring Team Handicap Differences into Marks

At the start of the first game, each team finds its handicap. The team handicaps are then compared to determine the pin difference, if any.

Should one team have 6 or more pins handicap than the other, the difference is converted into marks (i.e., the difference is divided by 10). This number of marks is then recorded on the lower left edge of the scoresheet to indicate the advantage one team has at the start of the game.

Cumulative marks are then recorded for each game in each frame to allow the teams to see their competitive progress throughout the game. In this way, a team can tell how far ahead or behind they are at the end of any given frame.

In figuring marks from the handicap, if the figure comes out to a fraction, round it off to the closest number. This is the only time any numbers are rounded off. In all cases of figuring averages and/or handicaps, any extra pins or fractions are dropped.

Mark Chart for Various Game Scores

The following chart indicates how many marks (strikes and spares) are normally required to reach different scores. A maximum score of only 90 is possible without making a spare or strike. And, it is impossible to bowl over 200 without having two strikes together.

To Score:	Marks Required:
91-103	1
104-113	2
114-123	3
124-133	4
134-143	5
144-153	6
154-163	7
164-173	8
174-183	9
184 & Over	10

Absent League Bowler

Each league establishes a "blind score" or "dummy" score in case a member of a team is absent. The most commonly used "blind score" is found by taking the absent bowler's current average minus 10, which is his or her game score. By using the aforementioned "mark chart," the team may place in "marks" according to the "blind score" in order to keep the mark count accurate.

Setting Up A League Schedule

In setting up a league schedule, the most important factor to consider is to make sure each team gets an equal chance. This is accomplished by making sure the teams rotate lanes each session and that each team gets to roll against all other teams an equal number of times.

Lane assignments can be assigned for the entire league schedule the first day of the league. The following are single round robin schedules for leagues with 6, 8, 10, or 12 teams, respectively.

League Lane Assignments

6 Team Schedule
Insert Lane Numbers

DATE			
	Team Code Numbers		
1	1-2	3-4	5-6
2	3-5	2-6	1-4
3	1-6	2-3	4-5
4	4-2	1-5	6-3
5	6-4	1-3	5-2

League Lane Assignments   **8 Team Schedule**

Insert Lane Numbers

DATE				
	Team Code Numbers			
1	1-2	3-4	5-6	7-8
2	6-8	5-7	2-4	1-3
3	5-4	1-8	7-3	2-6
4	3-6	7-2	1-5	8-4
5	7-1	4-6	3-8	5-2
6	2-3	8-5	4-1	6-7
7	4-7	6-1	8-2	3-5

League Lane Assignments   **10 Team Schedule**

Insert Lane Numbers

DATE					
	Team Code Numbers				
1	1-2	3-4	5-6	7-8	9-10
2	7-3	1-6	2-9	5-10	8-4
3	4-5	9-8	10-1	3-2	6-7
4	9-1	5-3	4-7	8-6	10-2
5	10-7	6-2	8-3	4-1	5-9
6	5-8	10-4	7-2	6-9	1-3
7	6-4	7-9	1-5	10-3	2-8
8	3-9	8-1	6-10	2-4	7-5
9	8-10	2-5	9-4	1-7	3-6

League Lane Assignments   **12 Team Schedule**

Insert Lane Numbers

DATE						
	Team Code Numbers					
1	1-2	3-4	5-6	7-8	9-10	11-12
2	4-5	6-2	12-3	9-11	1-7	10-8
3	9-3	1-10	11-4	5-12	8-2	6-7
4	7-12	5-8	9-2	10-4	11-6	1-3
5	11-8	9-7	1-5	6-3	10-12	2-4
6	10-6	11-1	3-8	12-2	7-4	9-5
7	5-7	4-12	2-10	1-9	6-8	3-11
8	12-9	10-5	7-11	4-6	2-3	8-1
9	6-1	2-11	8-12	3-5	4-9	7-10
10	3-10	8-9	4-1	2-7	5-11	12-6
11	8-4	7-3	6-9	11-10	12-1	5-2

Appendix C

Rules of Bowling

The following is a summary of rules and regulations in the game of bowling as established by the American Bowling Congress and the Women's International Bowling Congress:

- In league play, a team shall start bowling on the lane for which they are scheduled. The team then alternates lanes with the paired lane for each succeeding frame. The second game is started on the paired lane.
- A ball is legally delivered when it leaves the bowler's possession and crosses the foul line into playing territory.
- During or after the delivery, if any part of a bowler touches beyond the foul line, it constitutes a foul. The following are other interpretations concerning fouls:

  1. Touching a wall, post, or other structure, unless local ground rules are established, also constitutes a foul.

  2. When any foreign object drops from a bowler (i.e., keys, cap, jewelry, pens, and so on) on or across the foul, the bowler should signal the scorer or opposing team before picking up the dropped article to avoid any possibility of being charged with a foul.

3. If the bowler's hand or any other body part touches the lane beyond the foul line, a foul must be called. This is true even if the foul detecting device did not register the foul.

4. If the bowler's foot (or any other part of the body) crosses the foul line on an adjacent lane, a foul must be recorded.

5. A foul cannot be called when the ball rolls over the foul line during delivery.

6. A foul is not committed when a bowler crosses the foul line but retains possession of the ball.

- If a bowler fouls on the first ball delivery of a frame, the pins knocked down do not count and all of the pins are reset for the second ball delivery. Only the pins knocked down on the second ball roll count. If a bowler does knock all 10 pins down with the second ball, it is recorded as a spare.
- If a bowler fouls on the second ball of a frame, only the pin count from the first ball roll is recorded.
- Pins knocked down by a ball that first falls into the channel do not count. If this occurs on the first roll of a frame, this pin(s) must be reset before the next ball delivery.
- Pins that are moved off to the side or bounce off the lane and

back again, but remain standing, are considered as pins standing. If any standing pin is knocked down by the pinsetter, it must be placed into position before the next ball roll.

- All deadwood (pins knocked down) must be cleared from the lane before the next ball is delivered.
- Pins knocked over by a ball rebounding off the rear cushion do not count.
- In the case of a "dead ball," that ball shall not count and the pins shall be respotted for a rebowl situation. The following are situations where a "dead ball" is declared:

  1. There is interference with the ball before it reaches the pins.

  2. One or more pins are missing from the set-up.

  3. Bowling on the wrong lane or out of turn.

  4. When a player is interfered with before the delivery is completed, providing the bowler immediately calls attention to the fact.

  5. A pin is interfered with before the ball reaches it.

Appendix D

History of Bowling

Bowling may very well be the oldest form of recreation in the world today. An ancient version of a ball and pins resembling the current day bowling equipment was found in an Egyptian child's grave dating back to approximately 5200 BC More than likely the Stone Age man may have enjoyed rolling rocks at other rocks. We know the ancient Polynesians played a game resembling bowling in which they used pins and balls made of stone and rolled the balls a distance similar to the length of the present lane bed.

It has also been recorded that about the time of Christ, rolling rocks down hills was a form of war maneuver used to bowl the enemy over with a strike. This skill was practiced by the soldiers in order to develop accuracy, and before long they found it to be a form of play. The Italian game of *bocce* (which is still widely played among persons of Italian descent) probably originated from this early war game.

The modern form of bowling at pins probably originated in ancient Germany, not as a sport but as a religious ceremony. The parishioner would bring his *"kegel"* and place it at the end of a cloister in the cathedral. He was then given a round stone to roll at the *kegel* which represented *"heide,"* the heathen. If the parishioner was successful in knocking down the *kegel,* he was to have cleansed himself of sin. According to a nineteenth-century German historian, Wilhelm Pehle, this religious ceremony had its origin as early as the third or fourth century, and lasted less than two centuries.

As time passed, the game of bowling evolved into a recreational pastime rather than a religious ceremony. Martin Luther is said to have enjoyed the game of bowling and built a bowling lane for the younger members of his family. He is also credited with establishing the first set of rules for ninepin bowling. In ninepin, the pins were set in a diamond shape with the kingpin in the middle. The object was to knock down as many pins as possible without spilling the kingpin.

The game of ninepin was the form of bowling which was brought to America by the Dutch early in the seventeenth century. One of the early playing areas was in lower Manhattan, the spot still known as Bowling Green.

The game of bowling flourished in America and spread throughout the states. By the mid 1830s, it became a gambling sport which led to legislation banning ninepins in the 1840s. In order to circumvent the legislation, a tenth pin was added and all of the pins were placed in an equilateral triangle.

The new tenpin game did suffer in some areas from gambling but the biggest hindrance was the lack of uniform rules and equipment specifications. In 1895, the American Bowling Congress (ABC) was organized to standardize the playing rules and regulations. By the early 1900s, women became very interested in the game of bowling and formed their own organization to standardize the rules and sponsor competition. The Women's National Bowling Association, today known as the Women's International Bowling Congress (WIBC), was formed in 1916.

Another stabilizing influence came in 1932 with the formation of the Bowling Proprietors Association of America (BPAA). This organization was designed to improve the management of the sport and to stimulate the growth of bowling throughout the country through promotion programs and tournament sponsorship.

During World War II, bowling became a widespread recreational sport. It was one of the leisure activities provided by the armed forces for the many soldiers in training as well as for wounded veterans. In 1943, the National Bowling Council (NBC) was formed to coordinate all phases of bowling in the war effort. After the war, NBC became an informational clearing house and legislative liaison organization for the sport. For many years, the NBC served as national coordinator for the sport of bowling.

Bowling attracts millions of participants. With the addition of new, attractive bowling centers with automatic pinsetting and scoring machines, bowling has become a family sport. By 1970, the nation's most popular indoor participation sport was being enjoyed by nearly 52 million Americans of all ages.

Appendix E

Glossary of Terms

ABC—American Bowling Congress; a bowling governing organization.

Alley—The 60 feet of pine and maple in front of the foul line on which the ball is rolled (more commonly known today as the lane).

Anchor Man—The last or fifth man in a team's line-up.

Angle—A combination of the direction of the delivery and the path the ball takes toward the pins.

Approach—Maple area behind the foul line where bowler executes steps and delivery.

Arrows—Aiming targets embedded in the lane to help a bowler align the starting position on the approach with the ball path down the lane.

Average—Figure reached by dividing the total sum of game or scores by the number of games bowled in one session or season.

Baby Split—Any split where the ball must be rolled in between, 2–7, 3–10, 4–5, 5–6, 7–8, or 9–10.

Backup Ball—A reverse hook; a ball that curves from left to right on the lane (for a right hander).

Bed Post—The 7–10 split.

Big Four—The 4–6–7–10 split.

Blind Score—Score given a team for its absent member.

Block—The application or build-up of oil in the center of the lane which, illegally, helps guide the ball to the pocket.

Boards—Individual strips of wood which make up the lane and approach.

Body English—Physical gyrations after the ball has been delivered, as if to steer the ball.

BPAA—The Bowling Proprietors Association of America; association of bowling center operators.

Break Point—The place on the lane (about 45 feet from the foul line) where the ball begins its hook.

Bridge—The distance between the finger holes.

Brooklyn Strike—A ball crossing into the 1–2 pocket resulting in a strike (right handers).

Bucket—The 2–4–5–8 and 3–5–6–9 leaves.

Channel—Accepted term for the gutter.

Cherry—To chop; to miss a pin of a 2-pin spare.

Chop—Picking a cherry.

Clean Game—A game with a mark in every frame.

Conditioner—The oil or dressing applied over the surface of the lane to prepare it for play.

Crossover—A ball going to 1–2 pocket side for a right hander, 1–3 for a left hander.

Curve—A ball which moves to the left from the moment it is delivered. Not a hook which waits until it nears the pins before breaking to the left.

Cushion—Barrier at the rear of the pit that absorbs the pins and balls.

Dead Ball—A ball with very little action; little pin carry.

Deadwood—Pins left down on pin deck after the first ball of a frame.

Deck—Portion of lane where the pins are set.

Decks (Pin Decks)—The area of the lane where the pins are placed.

Double—Two consecutive strikes.

Double Pinochle—The 4–6–7–10 set-up.

Dutch 200—A 200 game scored by rolling alternate frames of spares and strikes.

Error—A miss.

Fast—Lanes which hold down the hook; sometimes referred to as "oily" or "slick." Today these lanes are more accurately referred to as "holding."

Flip—Extreme delay in the motion of ball; right-to-left association with reactive resin bowling balls.

Foul—The act of going beyond the foul line as you deliver the ball.

Frame—one-tenth of a game.

Full Hit—A ball that hits squarely on the head pin. Used to describe any ball that hits the target squarely or dead center.

Full Roller—A hook type of release in which the thumb rotates 10 to 11 o'clock and fingers lift through the ball for a right hander.

Goal Posts—The 7–10 split.

Grave Yard—The toughest lanes on which to produce good scores.

Gutter—Channel on each side of the bowling lane.

Handicap—Adjustment in score totals between individuals or teams to equalize competition.

Head Pin—The number 1 pin.

Heads—The first 15 to 17 feet of the lane onto which the ball is released, made of maple.

High Hit, Heavy Hit—A strike ball that comes into the head pin more than the 3 pin of the 1–3 pocket.

Hook—A ball that breaks from right to left well after release (for right handers).

House Ball—A ball provided by the bowling center for customer use.

Kickback—Side partitions between lanes at the pit end.

King Pin—The 5 pin.

Lane—Sixty-foot maple-pine or synthetic surface in front of the foul line on which the ball is rolled; also called alley.

Leadoff—The first person on a team.

League—An organized group of teams competing on a regular, formal basis under a specific code of rules and regulations.

Leave—The pins left standing after the first ball has been rolled.

Lift—Giving the ball an upward motion with the fingers at the point of release.

Light Hit, Thin Hit—Strike ball that fails to come up into the 1–3 pocket; hits more on the 3 pin than the head pin.

Line—The path of the ball from release point to the pocket.

Locator Dots—The 3 rows of dots on the approach.

Lofting—Throwing the ball out on the lane well beyond the foul line so it drops from a height.

Mark—A strike or a spare.

Miss, Error, Blow—Ball not making contact with any pins standing.

Mixer—A good working ball that produces lively action among the pins.

NBC—The former National Bowling Council; bowling industry promotion and service organization.

Oil—The substance used to coat or dress the lanes.

Open Frame—A frame without a strike or spare.

PBA—Professional Bowler's Association; organization of male professional bowlers.

Perfect Strike—A ball that hits the pins squarely in the pocket (between the 1 and 3 pins) and clears the deck of all pins.

Perfect Game—A 300 game consisting of 12 strikes in one game.

Picket Fence—The 1-2-4-7 or 1-3-6-10.

Pinspotter, Pinsetter—Automatic machine that picks up and sets the pins for the bowler.

Pit—Area at the end of the lane into which the pins fall.

Pitch—The angle in relation to the center of the ball at which the thumb and finger holes of a ball are drilled.

Pocket—The areas between the 1 and 3 pins; the strike zone.

Powerhouse—A very strong hooking ball that seems to tear the pins apart.

Pumpkin—The opposite of powerhouse.

Pushaway—The outward, downward thrust of the ball that puts the ball into motion.

Reactive Resin Ball—Bowling ball with tacky surface created by a polymer added to urethane which provides more grip of the ball to the lane.

Scratch—Use of actual scores and averages in individual or team competition; non-handicap bowling.

Semi-Roller—A hook type of release in which the thumb rotates counter-clockwise (11 to 10 o'clock) and the finger lift throws the ball.

Sleeper—A hidden pin; the 8 pin in the 2–8 setup.

Slow Lane—Double meaning term used in describing a lane which either resists a hook or assists it. Varies with geographical areas.

Sour Apple—The 5-7-10 split.

Span—The distance between the thumb and finger holes.

Spare—Knocking down all 10 pins in one frame with two rolls of the ball.

Spinner—A method of release that imparts an excessive counter-clockwise rotation of the thumb (11 to 7 o'clock).

Split—Two or more pins left standing after the first roll with a pin down immediately between or ahead of them (providing the #1 pin is down also).

Spot—A target guide on the lane used to aid the bowler in directing his or her ball; also term used to designate the handicap given another bowler or team.

Strike—Knock down all the pins with the first roll of the ball in a frame.

Strike Out—Three consecutive strikes in the 10th frame.

Sweep—The metal mechanism that cleans the pin deck after each delivery of the ball.

Tap—An apparently perfect strike hit that leaves the 8 pin standing.

Target Arrow—Aiming device located on the lane approximately 15 feet in front of the foul line. Also called range finder or marks.

Triple—Three strikes in succession. Also called a turkey.

Turkey—Three strikes in a row.

Washout—The 1-2-10 or the 1-2-4-10 spares.

WIBC—Women's International Bowling Congress; an organization of women bowlers.

WPBA—Women's Professional Bowling Association, organization of female professional bowlers.

Working Ball—Ball that moves with good rolling action, see Mixer.

YABA—Young America Bowling Alliance, an organization sponsoring bowling for youth.

Appendix F

Bowler's Analysis Chart (National Bowling Council)

NAME _____ LEFT HANDED ☐   RIGHT HANDED ☐

GRIP: CONVENTIONAL ☐   FINGERTIP ☐   SEMI-FINGERTIP ☐   OTHER ☐

SPECS: WEIGHT _____   TOP ☐   SIDE ☐   FINGER ☐

TRACK: FULL ROLLER ☐   SEMI-ROLLER ☐   SPINNER ☐   OTHER ☐

STANCE
COMMENTS

FEET: STRAIGHT TO INTENDED LINE   YES ☐   NO ☐
CLOSE ☐   FAIRLY CLOSE ☐   APART ☐   TOES TOGETHER ☐
LEFT FOOT AHEAD ☐   RIGHT FOOT AHEAD ☐

WEIGHT DISTRIBUTION:
MOSTLY RIGHT ☐   MOSTLY LEFT ☐   EVENLY DISTRIBUTED ☐

KNEES: BOTH BENT ☐   RIGHT BENT ☐   LEFT BENT ☐   STRAIGHT ☐

RELATIVE HEIGHT OF BALL:
CHEST HIGH ☐   WAIST HIGH ☐   KNEE HIGH ☐

ALIGNMENT OF BALL:
RIGHT OF SHOULDER ☐   IN LINE WITH SHOULDER ☐
AT CENTER LINE ☐   BETWEEN SHOULDER AND CENTER LINE ☐

WEIGHT OF BALL:
RIGHT HAND ☐   LEFT HAND ☐   DISTRIBUTED BETWEEN BOTH HANDS ☐

ELBOW: TUCKED INTO HIP ☐   AWAY FROM HIP ☐

WRIST: STRAIGHT ☐   FAIRLY STRAIGHT ☐   BENT ☐

THUMB POSITION: RELATIVE POSITION ON CLOCK _____

APPROACH COMMENTS

NUMBER OF STEPS _____

LENGTH OF STEPS: LONG ☐ MODERATE ☐ SHORT ☐

TEMPO: FAST ☐ MODERATE ☐ SLOW ☐

HEEL-TOE ☐ SHUFFLE ☐

STRAIGHT ☐ DRIFT RIGHT ☐

DRIFT LEFT ☐

ARMSWING: PARALLEL ☐ OUTSIDE-IN ☐ INSIDE-OUT ☐

LOOP ☐ BENT ELBOW ☐

RIGHT ANGLES TO INTENDED LINE:

SHOULDERS   HIPS

FACING { RIGHT ☐   FACING { RIGHT ☐

         LEFT ☐   LEFT ☐

BACKSWING: BELOW WAIST ☐ WAIST HIGH ☐

AT SHOULDER LEVEL ☐ ABOVE SHOULDER LEVEL ☐

WRIST: FIRM ☐ BENT BACK ☐ CUPPED ☐

BALANCE LINE: GOOD KNEE BEND ☐ TOO MUCH ☐ NOT ENOUGH ☐

GOOD WAIST BEND ☐ TOO MUCH ☐ NOT ENOUGH ☐

RELEASE COMMENTS

PALM: DOWN ☐ LEFT ☐ UP ☐ RIGHT ☐

WRIST: FIRM ☐ SAGGED ☐ ROTATES: . . LEFT ☐ RIGHT ☐

FINGERS: FIRM ☐ CLOSED ☐ OPEN ☐

LIFT: SMOOTH ☐ CRISP ☐ WEAK ☐

OUTSIDE FINGERS: BOTH CLOSE ☐ BOTH SPREAD ☐

INDEX FINGER SPREAD ☐ LITTLE FINGER SPREAD ☐

LITTLE FINGER TUCKED UNDER ☐

FOLLOW-THROUGH COMMENTS

DIRECTION RELATIVE TO TARGET:

IN LINE ☐ RIGHT OF TARGET ☐ LEFT OF TARGET ☐

HEIGHT:

WAIST ☐ SHOULDER ☐ OVERHEAD ☐ INCONSISTENT ☐

BALL ROLL COMMENTS

ACTION: STRAIGHT ☐ HOOK ☐ CURVE ☐ BACK-UP ☐

NUMBER OF BOARDS _____

HITTING POWER: STRONG ☐ WEAK ☐ NORMAL ☐

METHOD OF AIMING
COMMENTS

SPOT:	FOUL LINE ☐			LINE
	DOTS ☐	PIN ☐	SHADOW ☐	OR ☐
	ARROWS ☐			AREA

SPARE SHOOTING
COMMENTS

SPOT BOWLER: SPARE TO LEFT
    USES STRIKE TARGET—MOVES RIGHT ☐
    FOOT PLACEMENT SAME—TARGET MOVED ☐
    COMBINATION ☐
SPOT BOWLER: SPARE TO RIGHT
    USES THIRD ARROW—MOVES FEET LEFT ☐
    FOOT PLACEMENT SAME—TARGET MOVED ☐
    COMBINATION ☐

COMMENTS: 1st ANALYSIS	2nd ANALYSIS	3rd ANALYSIS	4th ANALYSIS

Index